Advance Praise for *Yoga for All of Us*

"*Yoga for All of Us* is an outstanding resource and exceptional guide to increased well-being and balance by one of this country's most accomplished yoga teachers."
—Angeles Arrien, Ph.D., cultural anthropologist, author of *The Second Half of Life*

"Peggy gives you a view of yoga expressly designed for those of us who never thought we could slow down enough to master it. She is a master, and she willingly shares her deep experience and wisdom."
—Beverly Kaye, founder/CEO, Career Systems International, coauthor *Love 'Em or Lose 'Em: Getting Good People to Stay* and *Love It, Don't Leave It: 26 Ways to Get What You Want at Work*

"For those of us who are getting on in age, whose sinews bind and joints creak—who think yoga is only for the tuned and flexible—Peggy Cappy's program can open us up to hope and vigor."
—Richard Meryman, author of *Andrew Wyeth: A Secret Life*

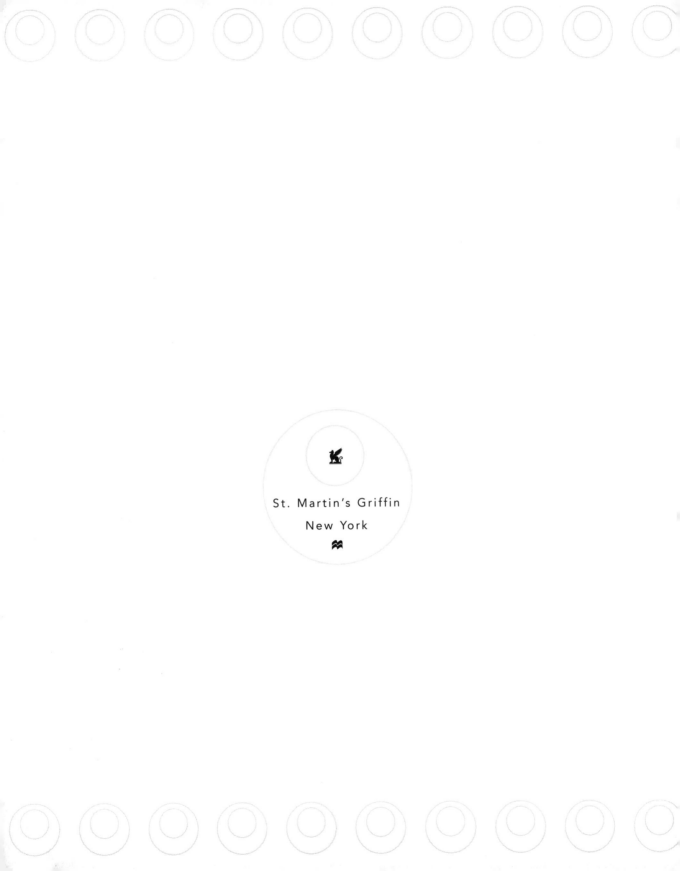

St. Martin's Griffin

New York

Yoga

FOR ALL OF US

A Modified Series of Traditional Poses for Any Age and Ability

PEGGY CAPPY

YOGA FOR ALL OF US. Copyright © 2006 by Peggy Cappy. Foreword copyright © 2006 by Laurie Donnelly. All rights reserved. Printed in the United States of America. No part of this book may be used or reproduced in any manner whatsoever without written permission except in the case of brief quotations embodied in critical articles or reviews. For information, address St. Martin's Press, 175 Fifth Avenue, New York, N.Y. 10010.

www.stmartins.com

Design by Susan Walsh

Photographs by Peter Wrenn

Library of Congress Cataloging-in-Publication Data

Cappy, Peggy.
 Yoga for all of us : a modified series of traditional poses for any age and ability /
Peggy Cappy—1st St. Martin's Griffin ed.
  p. cm.
 ISBN-10: 0-312-34087-7
 ISBN-13: 978-0-312-34087-2
 1. Hatha yoga. 2. Exercise for older people. 3. Exercise for middle-aged persons. I.
Title.

RA781.7.C357 2006
613.7'10846—dc22

2005045642

First Edition: April 2006

10 9 8 7 6 5 4 3 2 1

To the students of my Gentle Stretch Yoga Class:
Alice, Anne, Barbara, Betsey, Betty, Catherine, Christine, Dick, Dot, Duffy, Ed, Eve, Erika, Frank, Georgia, Gerry, Ginny, Ginty, Hank, Harriet, Janet, Jim, Jo, Joanne, Judy, Julie, Karen, Leandra, Lee, Lilla, Lisa, Lorraine, Mary Elizabeth, Mary Jane, Mimi, Priscilla, Robin, Ruth, Sidney, Susan, Ted, Tom

CONTENTS

FOREWORD

In early June of 2001, Peggy Cappy walked into my office at WGBH in Boston, Massachusetts, to present an idea she had for a television show. As a producer of lifestyle programming for public television, I see many ideas, but unfortunately we cannot produce all of them. In Peggy's case, however, I saw something unique—both for television and as a practice to be used beyond the lens. Peggy has been teaching a modified approach to yoga to a group of senior citizens for more than fifteen years, and the results for her class members are astonishing. By the end of the meeting and after reviewing some of her materials, I knew that WGBH had to partner with Peggy to bring her class *Yoga for the Rest of Us* to a broader audience.

By visiting with Peggy in Peterborough, New Hampshire, and taking one of her classes, I witnessed first-hand the Peggy Cappy difference. She is a gifted teacher. After watching the class, doing it myself, and then meeting with the extraordinary people she teaches, I understood that she was bringing a life-enhancing gift to those who might previously have thought physical exercise and yoga were beyond their abilities. I realized that in addition to producing a home video or "home class," we should also showcase some of the people whose lives had been changed by her yoga—in so doing, we would inspire others to try it. And we did.

Peggy has taught me and the thousands of people who have bought her videos and watched her on public television that by using Peggy's techniques, YOU CAN DO YOGA. Forget those same old excuses—I am too old; I am too far out of shape; I am too overweight; Yoga is for people who can bend like pretzels. Do yourself a favor and give Peggy Cappy's modified yoga a try.

Having worked with Peggy on both of her highly successful videos, I know what a change is in store for you. We have heard from many people, via e-mail and letters, about the benefits they have experienced from Peggy Cappy's approach to yoga.

Happy yoga . . . here's to positive changes and to feeling better.

—Laurie Donnelly
Executive Producer, Lifestyle Unit
WGBH Boston

ACKNOWLEDGMENTS

Many people have contributed significantly to the making of this book, directly or indirectly. I am deeply grateful and offer my heartfelt thanks to the following people:

All my students from every Gentle Stretch Yoga Class. I could not have done this book without our years together. Their trust in me, willingness to try every modification, and their generous and open hearts are a constant inspiration. I so appreciate their questions, stories, commitment to yoga, their well-being, and, most of all, the love we share.

My grandmother, Jean McTavish McPhail Wharff, whose quest for knowledge, fascination with Yoga and India, and eagerness to try new things was thankfully passed on to me.

My parents, Rosalie and Robert Zerkel, who honored my soul's uniqueness with boundless and abiding love.

My yoga and meditation teachers who have inspired and awed me with their knowledge and wisdom, I am indebted to each of them, whether my time with them was brief or over many years—particularly Swami Muktananda, Gurumayi Chidvilasananda, Jean Couch, Angela Farmer, Victor Van Kooten, Lilias Folan, Ana Forrest, Richard Freeman,

John Friend, Vyaas Houston, B. K. S. Iyengar, Judith Lasater, Aadil Palkhivala, Larry Payne, François Raoult, Kali Ray, Tracey Rich and Ganga White, Swami Satchidananda, Alexandra Teague, Thich Nhat Hanh, Sarala Troy, Janaki Vunderink, Patricia Walden, and Rodney Yee.

Laurie Donnelly for her enthusiasm and belief that my class "Yoga for the Rest of Us" would make great Public TV. And to the rest of the amazing people at WGBH in Boston, whose continued interest and support has been invaluable.

Patricia Nelson and Ike Williams at Fish & Richardson who have given their impeccable knowledge to this project.

Sheila Curry Oakes, Julie Mente, and all at St. Martins Press for the vision and hard work necessary to get my words to print.

Marian Lizzi for that first exciting phone call and her unwavering enthusiasm and belief that what had appeared on Public TV would make a good book. These pages would not be here without her.

The Women of Power and Grace, Melissa Stephenson and Lori Hanau, whose insight and laughter continue to nourish me.

Karen Johnson, for the hundreds of details she kept track of in helping the office run smoothly, including her dedicated customer support—she frees me to do the things I do best.

Debra Boudrieau, whose consummate skill as a writer, and whose absolute support as my closest friend, made her the perfect one who could craft this book with me. She knows my "voice" and without exception urged me to be true to it.

Alan Ebright, whose love and caring has brightened my life in untold, immeasurable ways (not the least of which is awesome technical expertise, which saved me countless hours of extra work).

All the people who made the photo shoot a fun and easy time, especially Peter Wrenn for his expert photography and his kind, patient, positive presence; Louise Daniels Miller, makeup artist extraordinaire, who is always attentive to every moment of any production; Alexandra Teague, whose discerning eye and knowledge of yoga coaxed the best poses out of us; the four yoga models—Josephine Day (100 years "young" as of May, 2006), Ted Dawes, Cathie Sage, and Kwame, who help show the world that indeed yoga is for the rest of us; and Dick and Liz Meryman, who generously turned over their home to be our yoga photography studio.

Mimi Bull and Anne Lunt, both members of the Gentle Stretch Yoga Class, who read through the manuscript and offered their supportive and insightful commentary.

Dick Meryman, for his encouragement to keep honing the words and for the gift of his writing expertise. His unexpected help has made all the difference in the first chapter of the book.

My extended family for their continued support over the years, Linda, Nancy, Jim, Em, and especially my daughter Leela and son Jason who "lived" yoga with me as they grew up, including traveling to India and embracing the austerities of a yoga and meditation community when other kids their age were enjoying the comforts of a "normal" life. . . . I love them beyond words.

Last, but not least, Isabelle Rosalie, my first granddaughter. May I be as inspiring to her growth as my own grandmother was to me.

INTRODUCTION

At this point in our human history, what was once reserved for
the most rare beings is available to ordinary people.
—Gangaji, an American-born spiritual teacher and author

I love yoga. I've been practicing it and teaching it for thirty-five years.
My hope for you is that once you have tried this modified and gentle
approach, you will love yoga just as I do. Or at least you will try it long
enough to experience its benefits.

If you have thought that the yoga you see depicted on the cover of
national magazines and on TV is not for you, you are probably right.
But my version of yoga is. I have modified a series of traditional poses
so that almost anyone can do them. The adaptations make each pose
accessible yet still offer the full benefits provided by the pose. For example,
I have added a chair to most poses to provide support as a safety for
balance work or, in essence to raise the floor eighteen inches to minimize the need for extreme forward bends.

If you are out of shape, over forty, recently recovering from an illness
or surgery, overweight, averse to gyms, with no classes nearby, or simply
a beginner who wants to start gently . . . this book is designed for you.

I think you'll be pleasantly surprised if you give yourself a month of
honest effort of doing a little yoga every day because I know that you
will see positive results. Yoga works. It has for thousands of years and

now it will for you because this program of modified poses can be done by almost anyone at any time. For instance, my grandmother.

One day when I was ten, I peeked into my grandmother's room. All I could see were feet and legs sticking up behind the bed. My curiosity got the better of me and I quietly made my way to where she was lying. I could see that she was in an upside-down position, resting on her upper back and head. I asked her what she was doing.

"I am doing my yoga. Do you want to join me?" my grandmother replied. It looked like fun. I got down on the floor beside her and soon I had my legs above my head in a position I now know as the Shoulderstand.

It was my grandmother's doctor who had recommended she try yoga for a temperamental back problem, and it worked. She found that by doing some yoga on a daily basis, she had no further trouble with back pain.

I loved my grandmother, everything from the look of her snow white hair to the feel of the soft skin on her arms. I liked spending time with her, but that summer when I was ten was the first time I had seen her do "her yoga."

As I grew older, I took pride in my grandmother's yoga skills. I loved to get her to demonstrate her agility. "Grandma, show me how you can touch the floor," I would plead. Obligingly she would bend forward from her hips and not only touch her fingers to the floor, but would place the flat of her palms to the outsides of her feet without bending her knees. I couldn't do that then, nor could any of my other family members.

My next significant exposure to yoga was in India, yoga's birthplace over five thousand years ago. When I was twenty-one, I spent several months traveling throughout India and Nepal. In India the practice of yoga is a total pursuit and a lifetime dedication, not an activity added to an already busy life, as we do it in America today.

In India one day I came upon several sadhus (saintly persons who practice yoga) meditating and doing yoga by a riverside. I was riveted by their ability to hold exotic poses for long periods of time. Wearing nothing but a loincloth, each was a sight. But I was most fascinated by what seemed to be their unwavering concentration when performing yoga. While one man sat unmoving in a seated meditation posture, another balanced endlessly on one leg in the Tree Pose.

I was intrigued by what I had witnessed in India and wanted to learn more. Returning to the United States in 1971, I immediately looked for instruction in yoga and meditation and found a yoga class offered by a wonderful teacher in the high school gymnasium, right there in my small New England town. I didn't know then how lucky I was. Yoga classes were then "few and far between." I wish I could remember my yoga teacher's name, but I will always remember her melodious voice and her gentle, careful guidance as I coaxed my eager body into foreign twists, stretches, and balancing poses.

As we did the Shoulderstand in that first class, I smiled because it was the pose my grandmother had shown me on the floor of her bedroom so many years earlier. But of all the poses that my teacher presented in my first class, I was most taken with the simplest and final one: the Pose of Relaxation.

My teacher turned the lights low at that point in the lesson, and her soothing voice guided me to a place of such contentment that my body seemed to be literally floating off the floor. Delicious currents of energy coursed through me. I wanted to stay as long as possible in that peaceful, blissful place. As the deep relaxation ended and my first yoga class was over, I had a flash of insight: I knew with an absolute certainty that yoga was something that I would do for the rest of my life.

After I had been taking yoga classes and studying meditation (yoga for the mind) for eight years, I wanted to share yoga with others through teaching. I was then—and still am—so enthusiastic about the enhanced well-being I experience from both yoga and meditation practice. I took my first yoga teachers' training in the summer of 1979 in upstate New York at a large meditation ashram—a place where a spiritual teacher instructs students in a sacred way of life.

The first classes I taught were in a small meditation center near my home. From the beginning I loved teaching. Word spread about my classes, and my enrollment increased quickly. To accommodate the numbers of students who wanted to benefit from yoga, I taught more and more classes. By 1982 I thought of myself as a yoga teacher and in the mid-1980s I opened my own yoga studio, which I operated for many years while continuing to study yoga. In the 1980s I returned to India and took my young children with me. For three months we lived in a yoga ashram where I obtained my advanced certification in teaching yoga and deepened my practice of meditation.

This book is based on a particular, weekly class ongoing since the late 1980s. Though I have been teaching yoga for over twenty-five years to diverse groups, this one became for me a kind of baseline, proof to me that anybody, willing to commit themselves, can improve their sense of well-being and improve their lives. I devoted myself to finding ways to give this lovely, heterogeneous collection of men and women that same peace and joy I had felt in my very first yoga class, the experience through which I knew yoga was for me—for the rest of my life.

The class members' ages range from forty to ninety-nine, so I modify classical yoga poses in dozens of ways to fit their capacities. For instance, to give them increased stability, I add a chair to the poses. Remembering a distracting chill I experienced in my first yoga class while lying on the drafty gymnasium floor, I provide blankets for my students. It's almost like tucking them in, preparing them for their relaxation experience at the end of class. My wish is to have all my students know the peaceful and joyful state of yoga, so that each will continue until they know for certain—yoga is for them, just like for me.

That wish is for you as well. Join me through the chapters that lie ahead. We'll create a yoga practice that works for you.

One

HOW TO USE THIS BOOK

Start where you are. Use what you have. Do what you can.
—Arthur Ashe, American tennis player

Begin now. Use this book daily. Set aside time to try these yoga poses, even just a little time. Leave this book out in a place where you can see it, and each time you see it, it will remind you to do yoga.

Pick a few things you want to work on and make a commitment to yourself to try them every day. If you want to improve your strength and stamina, practice a few of the standing poses each day. Try the same ones every day or vary your practice with a different set each time you experiment.

If you are looking for overall conditioning and a cardiovascular workout, the Sun Salutations alone make a wonderful addition to your day. Once you know them, you can do many repetitions in only five minutes (but set aside another couple of minutes for Relaxation to finish properly). Many of my students do that daily.

If you want a very gentle and easy way to limber up and a series of poses that combines breath with movement, try the entire Warm-up section. Once you know it, it will take you fifteen minutes and your whole body will feel great afterward.

Start where you want based on the changes you are looking for—

whether it's balance, strength, better breathing, or peace of mind, there's a chapter for each and more. It's the *doing,* and not just looking at this book, that will make *Yoga for All of Us* work for you.

Try to do some yoga every day. And there may be days when you can do much more than you usually have time for. The more you do, and the more often you practice, the more changes you will see. You will gain new physical skills as mentioned above and increase your mental abilities as well—like better concentration and focus. As you progress, select the poses and practices that challenge and inspire you; one day you might find that you are able to do a new pose or hold a pose longer than you ever dreamed possible.

THIS BOOK IS FOR YOU

I have designed this book so that just about anyone can do yoga. Instructions for each of the classical yoga poses include variations to simplify the poses. Use the modifications if you have physical limitations in balance, flexibility, or strength. If you are not very fit, start with the gentlest or easiest version.

Most of the yoga is designed to be used with a chair. Don't hesitate to use one. Using a chair will not decrease the effectiveness of this program. Rather it will help you maximize your results. For example, you will feel bolder when working on a balance pose if you know the chair is there to rescue you.

There are fewer yoga poses in this book than in many books on yoga. Of the hundreds to choose from, I have selected the classical ones that lend themselves to being adapted for a beginner's needs. I have not included any of the risky or extreme poses. There are no inverted poses and few backbends. I want you to have a safe and gentle introduction to yoga so you will experience its many benefits.

This book begins with gentle warm-up movements and stretches. Though they may not seem challenging, don't underestimate the significance of these simple starters. They are useful in getting you moving, increasing the range of motion in your joints, and improving circulation throughout your body. You will feel a "before" and "after" difference, like increased warmth in your shoulders or a good-feeling tingly sensation in your ankles and feet. After I do the side stretches, I am aware of the muscles between my ribs and know that even they have received some exercise. One of my students, a man in his eighties says the Warm-up series is like spreading "tiny bubbles of energy" throughout his body.

Strong on practical help in getting you started doing yoga safely, this book contains little yoga philosophy. There are many different approaches and schools of yoga and a profound and comprehensive philosophy. That can be fascinating once you have a practical understanding of yoga and want to place the poses in a philosophical context. For now, all you need is to get started. The esoteric framework can come later if and when you want it.

BEFORE YOU BEGIN

Check with your doctor before beginning the activities in this book if you have had a recent operation or injury, have restricted mobility, a chronic condition or complaint, or you are significantly overweight. There are certain disorders, like osteoporosis (low bone mass), that require special precautions to ensure safety in movement. If you are concerned, show this book to your doctor or knowledgeable therapist so that he/she can see its unique, gentle, and modified approach to yoga and understand what you are undertaking.

Please proceed with care and attention. Move out of any position that causes you pain or extreme discomfort. Your best approach is "easy does it." Don't push beyond your limits. Yoga does not endorse the "no pain/no gain" way of thinking.

Be aware that while the poses are deceptively simple, your appreciation and experience of them will change over time. A student named Barbara, who was new to yoga, said, "When I first started I thought *This can't be doing very much,* but I was very wrong." As Barbara found out, the most simple of poses have the power to transform body and mind.

Don't expect instant results, however. It has taken time for your body to get into the shape it is in now, and with time and practice you will be pleased at the well-being you can regain. The long-term benefits are immense.

The good news is that you don't need any special preparation to begin yoga. Occasionally potential students tell me that they will start yoga when they are in better shape or are more flexible, but I tell them not to wait. No matter how stiff you are, you can increase your flexibility with surprising speed. You'll also get stronger, gain better balance, learn to breathe better, and cultivate a calmer mind and a more resilient spirit.

WHAT YOU NEED

To get started all you need is this book, a chair, and a willing spirit. You can do yoga almost anywhere you have enough space to spread out and enough privacy to be comfortable. It is best to choose a strong, sturdy chair, like a kitchen chair, as an aid to your safety for the standing poses, but even a folding chair will do.

The use of a yoga mat—sometimes referred to as a "sticky mat"—under the chair is helpful because it provides a nonslip surface for both the chair and your feet. Make sure all four legs of the chair rest firmly on the mat to keep the chair from moving as you lean on it. If you have no mat, place the chair against the wall or a heavy piece of furniture so the chair will not slip away from you.

You don't have to use a mat to begin your practice of yoga, but yoga enthusiasts benefit by having a yoga mat. Not only do you create a nonslip surface, but by spreading out your mat, you create and define your yoga space.

> A fellow yoga teacher says, "The most difficult yoga pose is that first step onto your mat."
> *Judith Hanson Lasater, Ph.D., and physical therapist, yoga teacher since 1971 and author of 30 Essential Yoga Poses.*

WHAT TO WEAR

Wear clothing that is comfortable and not restrictive or binding. A T-shirt and leggings or a sweatshirt and sweatpants work fine. In the privacy of their homes, some people do yoga in their under garments.

Practice barefoot. Bare feet grip the floor or mat better and prevent slipping. Also, without socks or stockings, you will be aware of the muscles in your feet and feel how to use your feet effectively as a base of support in the standing and balancing poses.

WHEN TO DO YOGA

The best time of day to do yoga is simply the time that works best for you: morning, noon, or night. There is something positive to be said for each time of day.

Practice yoga in the morning, particularly if you feel stiff then—I have noticed that my dog and cat never fail to stretch after waking from the night's sleep. Try doing yoga before your regular daily activities begin. No time then? Get up a little earlier than usual. The benefit of fifteen or twenty minutes of yoga easily outweighs that much missed sleep.

Try yoga at noon. It may provide a welcome break in your day and help refresh and reinvigorate you for the afternoon.

Yoga in the evening or at the end of the day helps you to unwind and relieves weariness and muscular tension. Your body will be the most limber after a day's worth of activities, and stretching may be easier later in the day.

It is better to practice yoga before a meal rather than after. Bending and twisting the torso affects the internal organs like the stomach, as well as the muscles, nerves, and joints. You will feel more comfortable if you practice yoga on an empty stomach. If you need something to eat before your yoga time, have a glass of juice, a piece of fruit, or a very light snack. After a large meal it is best to wait several hours before doing yoga.

Set a time to practice and choose a place where you will be undisturbed by family members. Close the door on distractions. Turn off the phone and put e-mail on hold. Give yourself the time you deserve. Create a new habit of yoga by setting aside the same time in your day, every day. Yoga done every day will yield the best results. You will also see benefits if you practice only once or twice a week, just not as quickly. The more effort you put in, the greater the reward.

IN SILENCE OR WITH MUSIC?

Many yoga teachers and students relish silence while doing yoga. Much of the day is filled with noise and sound, so doing yoga may be the only time you experience silence. While practicing yoga in silence, you may become aware of noises that you normally tune out—the hum of a refrigerator or fan, the drone of traffic, the bark of a dog, or the melodious song of a bird. If those or other outside sounds are a distraction, use them as a reminder to shift your focus and turn your senses back to the task at hand: feeling the action and effects of each pose. Make each noise you hear an opportunity to refocus your awareness from the outer events to what is happening with your body, mind, and breathing.

As you listen to your body, you may become aware of your own breathing. A simple aid to help you hear the sounds of your inhalation and exhalation is inexpensive foam earplugs, which intensify the sounds of your breath. This and the breathing exercises (see Breathing, chapter

2) will show you how to use your breath as a powerful tool to link mind and body. Breath becomes a means to keep your mind focused on the present moment.

Some yoga teachers play music in their classes to minimize outside sounds. Others use music as a focusing devise. You may wish to play music as well. I often play music with a steady rhythm when I do many repetitions of Sun Salutation. I have used Pachelbel's *Canon in D* for many years in my classes for the Sun Salutations. The regular interval of notes helps set an even pace as we move through and repeat the pattern of the twelve positions of the Sun Salutation.

Music also can help you shift your energy and help you transition to the point when you can work with silence. For example, if you are tense, agitated, or keyed up when you start a yoga session, soothing music may help slow you down and assist in calming yourself more quickly. Then you can be more receptive to concentrating on your breathing and focusing on your inner being. Alternatively, if you are feeling lethargic, sluggish, or depressed, playing upbeat music at the start of your yoga session might give you a desirable boost to actually start you moving and doing yoga.

HOW TO PRACTICE

Once you have determined how long you have to practice, the length of time will dictate how many poses you can fit into the session. The number of poses will differ, of course, if you have thirty minutes for yoga rather than ten. One day you might decide to do all the poses of one type, like the Standing Balance poses, the Warm-ups, or the Sun Salutation series. On another, you could select one or two poses from each major grouping, moving in order from chapter 3 to chapter 9. The Relaxation Pose (chapter 11) should conclude every practice session, even if it is for only two to three minutes. Breathing (chapter 2) and Meditation (chapter 12) can be practiced anytime independently or as a part of your yoga practice time.

How do you decide? Take a few quiet moments and see what you are most drawn to do or what you are most attracted to or repelled by. Either might be the perfect place to start. When you are familiar with all the individual poses as well as the groups of poses, rely on your intuition to select the day's sequence.

During each session, take time to focus on your breathing and the sensations that the poses create. Be aware of how your muscles and joints feel in the poses and afterward, the quality of your breathing while you are working, and even emotions that arise unexpectedly.

Remind yourself to breathe through each pose. When beginning to learn yoga, many people have a tendency to hold their breath, particularly when they are concentrating hard, exerting effort, or striving to hold their balance. If you come out of a pose feeling winded or breathing hard, you can be sure that you were not getting the breath you needed.

Hold a pose as long as you can remain steady and comfortable. Start out holding each pose for a short time, a duration of two or three breaths in and out. As your endurance builds you may be comfortable in a pose for a half minute, a full minute, or even longer. Come out of a pose as you begin to tire or feel shaky.

Always end your practice with several minutes of deep relaxation to give your body and mind an opportunity to balance and integrate your efforts. Because this is important, familiarize yourself with Relaxation (see chapter 11) before you begin to practice.

Invite a friend or family member of any age to try the exercizes in this book with you. This creates an opportunity to have a good time together and deepens your connection with one another. Have one of you read the instructions and watch while the other tries and refines the poses. For the Relaxation Pose, you can really let go and relax completely if your partner reads the instructions to you. Take turns and switch roles.

Practice in a spirit of fun, good humor, and nonjudgmentally. Don't be hard on yourself or overly critical. The more room for improvement you see, the more quickly you will experience positive results with regular practice. Be accepting of your starting point, whatever it is. Although you may want to set a specific goal for yourself, like being flexible enough to bend over and touch your toes, yoga is not meant to be practiced in a competitive spirit. Do your best each day and know your best will not be the same from day to day. Your flexibility and endurance will vary, so don't be discouraged if you have trouble for a couple of sessions in a row. It is part of the path of progress to sometimes feel you are making rapid improvement and at other times feel you are stuck or losing headway. Do focus on your overall improvement and how you feel after a satisfying session.

How a pose looks on the outside is not as important as what you are experiencing. You might think that an advanced practitioner is the person who can perform the most extreme position or a very difficult pose. In reality an advanced practitioner is one who practices each pose, no matter how simple or difficult, to the limits of his/her ability and with full awareness plus a quiet mind and then brings that inner knowledge into the daily world. Awareness is what makes yoga so much more than physical exercise. If you want to strive for anything in yoga, strive for an increased ability to know yourself as you become more proficient with the poses, the breathing, and the meditation exercises, and bring that better understanding into every interaction and activity in your daily life.

It is natural to share your enthusiasm for this approach to yoga with others. After several months of doing the class "Yoga for the Rest of Us," one eighty-year-old man regained the vitality and mobility that he had feared was gone forever. To celebrate his achievement, his daughter had a special T-shirt made that said, "Body by Peggy." When he wears it, others invariably ask, "Who's Peggy?" which provides him an easy opening to talk about yoga and all that it has done for him.

WHAT YOU CAN EXPECT

You may feel tired the first few times after doing yoga. Don't be concerned; fatigue is a common side effect but it will pass. Usually that tiredness is a result of an internal cleansing enacted by the poses and overall is a good thing for your body. The poses compress and release the tissues, glands, and organs. That stimulates circulation throughout your body and help flush out stored impurities and toxins. I think that the effect of beginning yoga is like a good housecleaning in a long-neglected home. As you first start to sweep and clean, dust fills the air. When the flurry of activity is over, the air clears, order is restored, and the house looks and feels wonderful. Yoga has a similar benefit for your body.

A good remedy for this beginner's tiredness is to give yourself extra time to rest in the deep relaxation following the poses. Your body will have the time it needs to do its cleaning and elimination, just as extra sleep and rest are important to healing and renewal.

Chances are that you will feel good results from your very first attempt at doing yoga. The poses may be just what you need to stretch out the tightness in your lower back or to banish stiffness in your joints and bring about a greater ease of movement through your day. You may alleviate tension in your neck and shoulders. A noticeable benefit will include mind as well as body: you may feel calmer and be quieter mentally. You may notice that you seem less distractible and are better able to concentrate, feel less scattered, and be more focused. You may be like me after my first yoga class: you haven't figured out what specifically it is about doing yoga that's made you feel so good, but you do know you want to do it again soon. That feeling can be the start to a life-long practice!

Benefits of Yoga

These are a few comments about the longer-term benefits from my students who practice yoga regularly:

"I now have enough breath to go up a flight of stairs without getting winded."
"I walk more gracefully, and I stand with more poise."
"I found the peace of mind to help me through a time of grief."
"I can now get around without my walker."
"I surprised my family on vacation; I could walk everywhere, even with knee replacements and arthritis!"
"Unlike many of my friends, I don't have a stiff joint in my body."

Two

BREATHING

Sometimes the most important thing in a whole day is the rest
we take between two deep breaths.
—Etty Hillesum, writer and victim of the Holocaust (1914–43)

Breath is absolutely essential to life. You can go weeks without food, days without water, but only minutes without breath. In one day you breathe in and out more than twenty thousand times. Because your breathing is automatic, a function of your autonomic nervous system, you probably don't give it much thought unless you have a breathing problem, like asthma or emphysema, or you get pneumonia or bronchitis.

Yoga teaches you to be conscious of your breathing, to improve how you breathe, and to increase and strengthen your vital life energy, which is linked to your breathing.

Your health is affected by the quality of your breathing as much as it is by the amount of sleep and exercise you get and the quality of the food you eat. One of the most important and subtle benefits of yoga is learning how to breathe in a way that enhances your well-being. You can change the way you breathe to increase your vitality, add years to your life, and improve your overall health.

Although your breath is a function of your autonomic system, your breath and your mind have a close relationship. A single thought or emotional state can change your breathing pattern. For example, when you are under a lot of stress, your breathing becomes restricted and each breath is short and shallow because you use only the upper part of your lungs and chest to breathe. However, when you are relaxed, your breath is steady, smooth, and easy. You use a greater area of your lungs and breathe in a larger volume of air, which circulates more oxygen through the blood to the entire body. Increased oxygenation of your blood means that every organ, gland, tissue, nerve, and cell of your body is enriched and functioning at its highest potential.

Yoga breathing exercises will increase your lung capacity and help your mind become more focused. The first sign of improved breathing may be an enhanced feeling of well-being and increased physical energy. Once you learn to do these exercises, you will be able to do them almost anywhere, and the benefits will be immediate and welcome.

For these breathing exercises and while doing the yoga poses, breathe out of your nose if you can for both the inhalation and exhalation because the nose filters and warms the air that enters your body. If you notice yourself using mouth breathing during your practice of the yoga poses, stop and rest, waiting until your breathing quiets. Switch to nose breathing if you are able and remain focused on your breathing, making each breath fuller, deeper, and more conscious. Mouth breathing happens when you are out of breath, or not getting the air you need. If your nose is stopped up or clogged due to a cold or allergy, breathe as best you can.

The following five breathing exercises are safe and effective for beginners.

CAUTION: If you get dizzy, tense, or begin to feel bad, stop and rest. Relax and try again at another time. The point is to do the breathing exercises with ease and without strain.

BREATH WITH ARM MOVEMENT

This exercise deepens your breathing and gives you practice coordinating your breath with movement.

Palms Turned Outward

Stand with your arms at your sides—your palms naturally face inward. Rotate your wrists and arms outward. As they rotate, your palms face front and continue to turn outward to the sides.

Arms Overhead

Take a slow, deep breath in as you lift your arms up from your sides to an overhead position.

As you breathe out, lower your arms, palms face up, to your sides.

Continue lifting and lowering your arms four more times, coordinating the movement with each breath. Make your breath full and deep on the inhalation, and long and slow on the exhalation.

Return to your beginning standing position with your arms relaxed and be attentive to the effect of those five deep breaths.

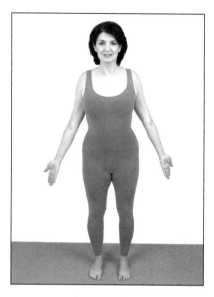

Palms Turned Outward

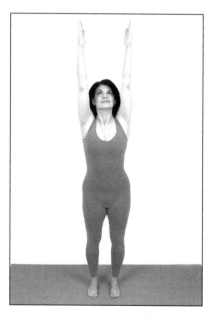

Arms Overhead

Belly Breathing, also called "the Abdominal Breath," is our natural, un-stressed breath. A baby naturally breathes this way. It's not until we are older that we tend to restrict our breath. Breathing from the belly is an efficient way to breathe and maximizes the entire area of the lungs because the incoming air is drawn down into the lower lobes.

This breathing exercise is best learned while lying down on your back. But once mastered, it can be done anywhere and at any time. A relaxed breathing style is the opposite of what commonly happens when you take a forced and deep inbreath by pulling in your belly and puffing out your chest.

Belly Breathing is the first step of the Three-Part Breath Exercise that follows. Practice Belly Breathing so that it is smooth and easy before attempting the Three-Part Breath.

Belly Breath, Abdomen Raised

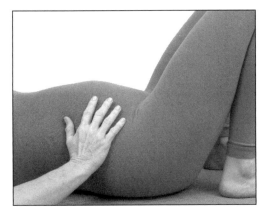

Belly Breath, Abdomen Raised

Take a slow, deep breath in and out with your breathing easy and free and your belly relaxed.

Place your hands on your belly below your navel.

Breathe into the area below your hands.

As you breathe in, expand your belly into your hands.

Belly Breath, Abdomen Lowered

As you breathe out, pull in your belly muscles slightly or simply let your belly relax down into your body.
Your belly rises and falls with each inhale and exhale.

Keep your ribs and upper chest quiet as you breathe.

Continue this breathing for 10 breaths or more.

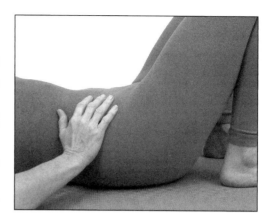

Belly Breath, Abdomen Lowered

This breathing exercise is so valuable that once you feel comfortable with it, you may want to extend your practice to five minutes at a time.

If it is difficult to feel the movement of your belly as it rises, you can bring your attention to your belly by placing a heavy book or a bag of rice below your navel. As you breathe in, move the object up, and as you breathe out, let it drop back down. Once you feel the movement of your belly in relation to your breath, remove the object and practice without it.

THREE-PART BREATH EXERCISE

This breathing exercise promotes the maximum expansion of your lungs, increases your breathing capacity, and recharges you, physically and mentally. I recommend a few repetitions of the Three-Part Breath Exercise after doing yoga poses or Sun Salutations (see chapter 10) once you lie down for relaxation (see chapter 11). This breathing exercise helps you relax quickly.

If you have awakened in the night and want to return to sleep, do ten or more repetitions of the Three-Part Breath. It is a comfort and an aid in going back to sleep because it promotes an immediate feeling of peace and well-being.

There are three parts to this exercise. Practice each part independently until you can do each.

1. **Belly Breathing**, (explained in the previous breathing exercise, see page 20).
2. **Rib-Cage Expansion**

   To feel the movement of your ribs, exhale completely and place your hands firmly against the sides of your lower ribs. Direct your attention to your hands as you breathe into your rib cage.

   As you breathe in, expand your rib cage. Feel your ribs move outward and separate.

   As you breathe out, contract your rib cage. Feel your ribs move in and together.
3. **Upper Chest Breathing**

   The movement of the upper chest is slight. To feel it, place your hand on your sternum and direct your attention to your hand.

   As you breathe in, raise your sternum (chest bone).

   As you breathe out, lower your sternum.

Combine the three breaths—belly, rib cage, and upper chest—into one long breath:

As you breathe in, fully expand the belly, then the ribs, and finally the upper chest, taking in the maximum amount of air. Note that once you begin to expand your ribs, your belly will pull in slightly.

As you breathe out, contract your belly all the way, then close your ribs and lower your upper chest in that order. Expel every bit of air.

Continue the Three-Part Breath for 10 complete breaths, counting an inhalation and exhalation together as one complete breath. Practice doing this breath work as a smooth and continuous movement for each inhalation and exhalation. Then, allow your breathing to resume its normal pace and rhythm.

ALTERNATE NOSTRIL BREATHING—*NADI SHODANA*
(NAH-dee SHOH-dah-nah)

This breathing exercise is calming and balances the hemispheres of the brain. At any given time, without being aware of it, you breathe mostly through one nostril, and it is usual for one side to be more open than the other. The dominance switches every two to two and a half hours and is controlled by your pituitary gland, which is considered to be the master gland of your body.

Learning the Alternate Nostril Breathing can be a little challenging, but don't let that stop you from trying it. The key to mastering it is to remember that whichever side you exhale from is the same side you inhale on. You will use finger placement to alternately block or unblock your nostrils, switching finger placement after each inhalation.

The finger position for Alternate Nostril Breathing:

Hand Position for Alternate Nostril Breathing

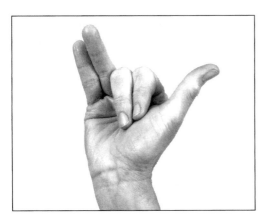

Make a loose fist with your right hand.

Extend your thumb and your fourth and fifth fingers (ring finger and pinky). Your other two fingers are curled against your palm.

This may feel awkward at first, but it is the traditional hand position used for this breathing exercise.

Take a deep breath in to completely fill your lungs.

Hand Position for Alternate Nostril Breathing

Thumb to Nostril

Begin the pattern of alternation as follows:
 Cover your right nostril with your right thumb.
Exhale slowly through your left nostril.
 Inhale slowly through that same side.

Ring Finger to Nostril

Close your left nostril with your ring finger as you re-lease your thumb.
 Exhale slowly though your right nostril.
 Inhale slowly through your right nostril.
 Repeat by covering your right nostril with your right thumb and exhale through your left nostril. Inhale through that same side. Switch sides.
 Continue by alternating the closing of each nostril. Consider one breath an exhalation followed by an inhalation on the same side.
 Practice for at least 2 minutes, but as much as 5 minutes if you are comfortable.
 Then sit or lie quietly for a minute to appreciate the mental clarity and quiet created by this breathing exercise.

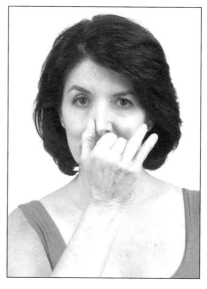

Thumb to Nostril

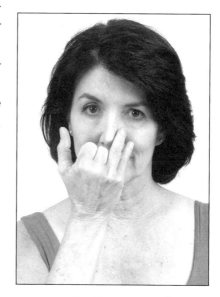

Ring Finger to Nostril

Some yoga poses have specific instructions for breathing, which I have included for each relevant pose. When there are no specific instructions given, follow these guidelines:

Breathe continuously when you are in the poses. Hold the pose and not your breath.

At all times be aware of the quality of your breathing. Take note of any time you are out of breath or breathing hard. That's a signal to stop what you are doing and allow your breathing to return to normal.

> The breathing exercises in yoga are known as *pranayama* (prah-nah-YAH-mah). According to Yoga, there is a subtle energy associated with the breath called *prana* (PRAH-nah), which means "breath." *Prana* is a body's life force or energy, and it exists in all living things. When the *prana* leaves a living being, the being dies. The *prana* runs through your body in currents called *nadis* (NAH-deez). *Nadis* comprise a network through which your body, mind, and spirit interact. *Pranayama* (*yama* means "regulation" or "control") is the practice in yoga whereby you strengthen your life force, make your nervous system healthy and resilient, and recharge your body with abundant energy.

Three

SEATED WARM-UP STRETCHES

I recommend being gentle with yourself . . . regardless of what
comes your way.
—Wayne Dyer, author and motivational speaker

While these exercises look simple and are simple, they are very valuable because they are very effective in stretching and warming your muscles, increasing the range of motion and flexibility of your joints and spine, enhancing the circulation in the specific areas of movement, and attuning yourself to your body's daily idiosyncrasies—joints and muscles that you might ignore but which also need your special attention due to tension, strain, injury, or disease.

An important aspect of these stretches goes beyond simply doing them. To fully experience the effect of the stretch in the part of your body you have been working, take a few moments when you are finished with each movement to stop and be still, attentive, and focused on that part of your body. For example, in the section on the neck and head, after you have completed the forward and backward head movement and have returned your head to its beginning position, feel the sensation in your neck created by the movement. You may perceive this as warmth, energy, or tingling because you have increased circulation to the area and have warmed the muscles through stretching them. The effect may be subtle so that you'd miss it without looking closely. When you look for and become aware of the effects, you will appreciate the benefits of these Warm-up Stretches. Knowing and appreciating the value of these stretches will help you make a regular place for them in your daily life.

These gentle stretches, drawn from my background in dance, are a great way to begin a yoga session. During my teens and twenties I studied dance, and each class always began with warm-up movements to prepare the body for more intense activity. It makes good sense to gently coax a stiff body into movement before more demanding work, so I begin each yoga class with stretches like these to prepare the body for the more challenging yoga poses.

There are two ways you can do these Warm-up Stretches: sitting in a chair or seated on the floor.

If you are comfortable in a cross-legged position on the floor, then start there. If the words comfortable and cross-legged just do not go together in your mind, use a chair. You will gain all the benefits of the movements whether you use a chair or do them on the floor.

If you choose to use a chair, pick a sturdy one with a hard seat and firm back, like a kitchen chair. A firm seat will give you more support than a cushioned or upholstered seat. If you are in a wheelchair, these stretches can be done from there.

The Warm-up Stretches are particularly useful on days when you have a long practice time of forty-five minutes to an hour, as you would in a class. They are not necessary before practicing a few yoga poses, but are a comforting way to begin a longer session.

You can also use these Warm-up Stretches without progressing to any yoga poses. Do them first thing in the morning as a great start to your day to enliven your body. Or you may want to use them at the end of your day as a way to release any accumulated muscle tension.

Once you have learned these gentle Warm-up Stretches, there is another way to use them: look for opportune places to add them in small doses to your daily routine. For example, make the foot movements before you get out of bed in the morning as you are waking up. Exercise the arms and hands during the commercials whenever you watch TV. Perform the head and neck movements when sitting down to take a break with a cup of coffee or tea. The next time you are stuck in traffic or at a traffic light, take the opportunity to do finger and wrist stretches one hand at a time. Anytime you can, remember to add some of the stretches to your day. Do these stretches and not only will your body benefit—if you pay attention to the sensations of the stretches while you are doing them, you will focus on the present moment and take a short break from thinking of the many distractions that can run around in your mind. I like to think of it as a minivacation for your mind.

Once you have increased your hip flexibility, you may be able to sit on the floor, at least for a few minutes at a time. Why should you bother trying this? Sitting on the floor helps to strengthen your back muscles and increases their ability to hold you upright with ease. I recommend that you practice sitting on the floor each day, even if it is just to slide off your couch or comfortable chair and onto the floor while you are watching TV or reading. If your back muscles are not strong enough yet to hold you up with ease, use the back of the sofa or chair to lean against. Start with your legs in a cross-legged position. When your legs get uncomfortable, relax them by stretching them out in front of you and gently massage them. Then pull them back in and switch the cross of your legs. Over time you will build up the ability to sit cross-legged comfortably.

Another terrific benefit of getting down on the floor is the practice in getting back up. As members of my seniors' yoga class will tell you, it is good to practice getting up from the floor. The day may come when you need that ability, and you'll be able to respond with grace and agility.

These stretches are simple and effective for loosening the tightness and stiffness in the neck area and working out occasional kinks. If you do these stretches on a regular basis, you will increase the range of motion in your neck and head area, and you will notice that certain actions will be easier, like looking over your shoulder to back up the car. A student of mine who suffers from tension headaches also finds relief by doing these stretches as part of her daily routine.

You can quickly do a set of these stretches anywhere—at your desk, in the car, or sitting and watching the news. Once you know these stretches, use them any time you feel that your neck muscles have become tense.

You may hear a crackly or gravel-like sound as you move your neck, particularly when you move from side to side. Don't be alarmed; although it may sound strange, it is not unusual. Despite how loud it may seem to you, it is an internal sound that can't be heard by anyone else in the room.

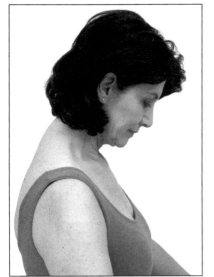

Head Forward

•

Head and Neck, Down and Up

Sitting in a chair or on the floor, take a full, deep breath in.

Head Forward

On the exhalation, gently drop your head forward and down, bringing your chin toward your chest. Feel the stretch in the back of your neck.

Head Up

On the inhalation, gently raise your head. Slowly lift your

nose and chin toward the ceiling. Feel the stretch this creates in your throat. Keep your jaw loose and relaxed. Your jaw will remain relaxed if you keep your teeth apart.

Repeat the basic movements up and down at a pace that is comfortable for you.

With each breath out, move your head forward and down,

With each breath in, move your head up and back.

After you have stretched at least five times in each direction, return your head to its neutral, upright position.

Take a moment to feel the sensation in the front and back of your neck as a result of the movement. You may feel a pleasant tingle or warmth in your neck muscles.

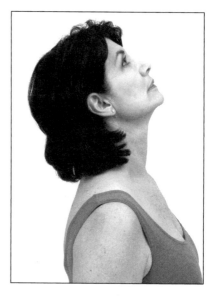

Head Up

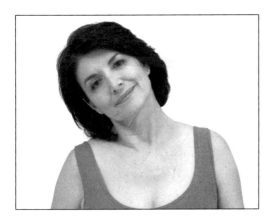

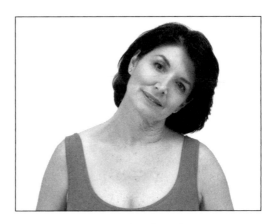

Head to the Right   Head to the Left

Head and Neck, Side to Side

Take a deep breath in.

Head to the Right

As you exhale, tilt your head to the right, dropping your right ear toward your right shoulder. Become aware of the stretch in the left side of your neck.

As you inhale, return your head to center—your neutral, upright position.

Head to the Left

Exhale as you drop your left ear toward your left shoulder, stretching the right side of your neck. Inhale and come back to center.

Repeat the basic movement from side to side, doing the movement in rhythm with your breathing—exhale as you move your ear toward your shoulder and inhale each time you come back to center.

YOGA FOR ALL OF US

Continue for at least 5 repetitions and end with your head in an upright position.

Take a moment to feel the sensation in the sides of your neck as a result of this movement.

•

Head and Neck, Turn from Side to Side

Begin with a deep breath in.

Head, Turn Right

As you exhale, slowly turn your head to the right side, moving your chin toward your right shoulder.

As you inhale, return your head to center,.

Head, Turn Left

Exhale as you turn your head to the left, moving your chin toward your left shoulder.

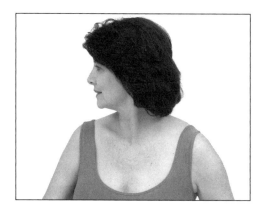

Head, Turn Right

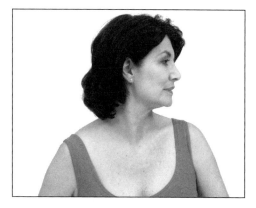

Head, Turn Left

SEATED WARM-UP STRETCHES

Inhale as you move back to the center.

An alternate breathing pattern for this stretch: exhale as you move to one side and inhale as you move to the other, not stopping in the center. Do the breathing this way if you want to move from side to side more quickly than using a separate inhalation and exhalation to each side. Repeat the basic movement with the breathing pattern that suits you best.

Move into the stretch a little farther each time you turn your head.
    Go to each side at least 5 times.
    Finish by bringing your head back to center.

Once you have completed these stretches, sit still for a moment. Focus your attention on your entire neck area to be aware of the sensations that these exercises have created.

Take a moment to name the sensations you are feeling. Does your neck feel warmer and softer—more like marshmallow and less like rock? Part of doing yoga is developing a greater understanding and awareness of how your body works and feels. If you start developing the skill of listening to your body now while doing these simple stretches, when you get to the yoga poses you will be more aware of how your body moves and feels and have had practice naming the sensations created by movement.

There is a Chinese saying that the secret to a long and healthy life is a flexible spine. The gentle movements of the torso in these exercises will loosen up your spine and add years of flexibility to your backbone. They will also stretch and lengthen the muscles of your torso and improve your posture.

When your posture is correct, the muscles of your back are in balance, remaining relaxed and with just enough muscular tension to hold your spine upright. Too much tension in the back causes the muscles to stay tight, creating bad posture and often resulting in pain. If you spend a lot of time sitting in a chair, or do a job that involves a lot of standing, or hold stress in your back, these stretches will help relax your back, ease your discomfort, and correct your posture.

Good posture not only looks and feels better, it causes your body to function better as well. Your lungs expand more, and you can breathe more fully when your body is not slouched. The performance of other internal organs is also improved. Students have remarked that these stretches make them feel more vital and alert. When energy and circulation are not restricted by tight muscles, both flow freely throughout the body and supply abundant oxygen and nutrients to the cells while effectively removing impurities and toxins. These three simple spinal movements will do much to improve your posture.

Yoga student Jo demonstrates the chair position.

CAUTION: If you have a spinal injury or a problem like osteoporosis, consult a health-care professional for guidance.

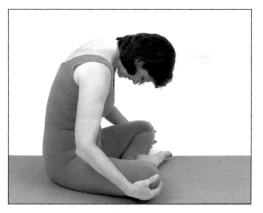

Forward Bend, Cross-legged Pose

Forward Bend and Spinal Extension

Forward Bend, Cross-legged Pose/Forward Bend, Chair

Sit in a cross-legged position on the floor, or in a chair with your spine upright and knees apart. Place your hands on your knees.

Begin by taking in a deep breath.

As you exhale slowly, bring your head forward, dropping your chin toward your chest.

Roll your shoulders forward and round your back as you lower your head toward your knees.

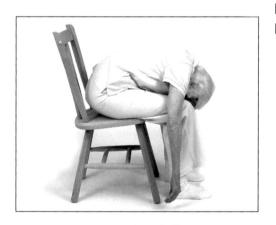

Forward Bend, Chair

Spinal Extension, Cross-legged Pose/Spinal Extension, Chair

As you inhale, uncurl your spine and return to an upright position.

With your hands around your knees, pull against them to help lift and extend your spine upward.

Pull your shoulders back and down, opening the front of your chest.

Gently lift your breastbone (center of your chest) to open up your chest farther.

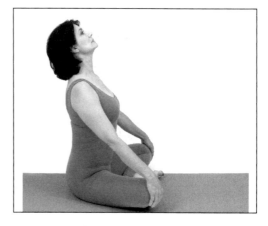

Spinal Extension, Cross-legged Pose

Repeat the basic movement with the breathing if possible. On an exhalation, round your spine forward; on the inhalation, uncurl, lift your spine, and expand your chest.

If you need or want more time to move than one breath allows, feel free to modify the breathing in this exercise. Take the number of breaths that is necessary.

Remain aware of each breath in and out, while also being attentive to the movement in your body.

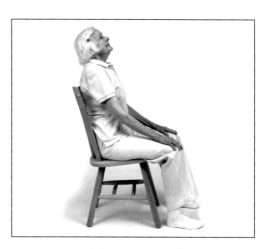

Spinal Extension, Chair

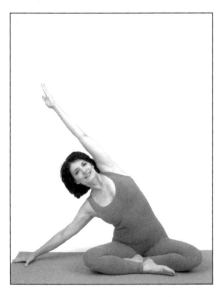

Side-to-Side Stretch, Cross-legged
Pose, Arm Raised

Side-to-Side Stretch, Cross-legged
Pose, Bend to the Right

Side-to-Side Torso Stretch

Side-to-Side Stretch, Cross-legged Pose, Arm Raised

Sit in an upright position. As you take in a deep breath, lift your left arm overhead, palm facing right.

Raise your fingers to the ceiling and stretch your entire left side, including your armpit, ribs, and waist.

Side-to-Side Stretch, Cross-legged Pose, Bend to the Right

As you breathe out, bend your torso to the right and stretch your left hand to the right.

Come back up to center.

Side Stretch, Chair, Arm Raised

Inhale as you lower your left arm and at the same time, raise your right arm overhead, stretching your right side from your fingertips to your waist.

Side Stretch, Chair, Bend to the Left

Exhale and bend your torso to the left, reaching across to the left side with your right arm.

Repeat the basic movement from side to side at least 5 times, focusing on your breath and the movement.

Each time you repeat the basic movement, increase the stretch, but stretch only as far as is comfortable.

Return to your neutral, upright position.

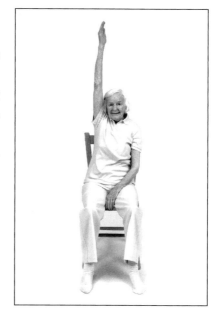

Side Stretch, Chair, Arm Raised

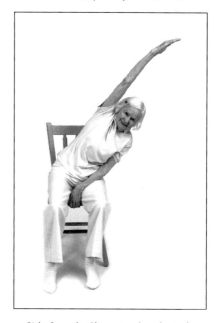

Side Stretch, Chair, Bend to the Left

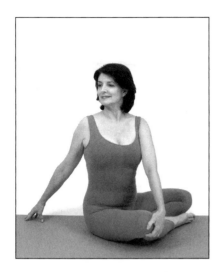

Spinal Twist, Cross-legged Pose

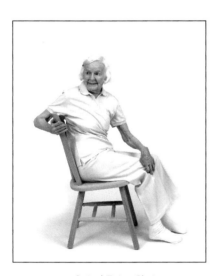

Spinal Twist, Chair

Spinal Twist

This Spinal Twist gives a gentle massage to your lower back and may help relieve minor backaches by aligning the spine. Also the twisting motion helps digestion and is beneficial for troubles with constipation.

Spinal Twist, Cross-legged Pose / Spinal Twist, Chair

Sit upright and place your right hand on your left knee as you take a deep breath in.

Move your left arm behind you to the back of the chair (or to the floor if seated cross-legged).

Exhale as you slowly turn to the left. Pull your abdominal muscles in and to the left as you twist.

Release the stretch and return to center as you inhale.

Repeat the stretch on the other side.

Repeat the basic movement on both sides twice more.

On the third time, hold the rotated position for several breaths on each side. As you breathe in, elongate and lift your spine. As you breathe out, pull the belly muscles around to that side and gently deepen your twist.

Return to center and take a deep breath in and out.

Take a moment to feel the sensations that these three Spine and Torso Stretches have created. Describe the feeling as best you can. One of my students refers to a champagne feeling that a good stretch brings.

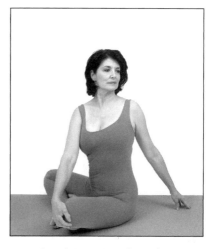

Spinal Twist, Cross-legged Pose

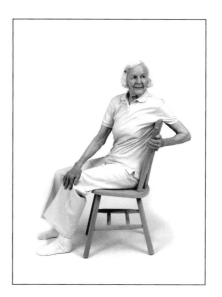

Spinal Twist, Chair

Your shoulders are another area where you can hold tension due to stress. These stretches not only loosen the shoulder joints, but are also a good remedy for stiffness in the muscles of the shoulders and upper back. The shoulder circles help to stretch and loosen the muscles that run between the shoulders and the breastbone, which helps keep the chest open and promotes a better posture.

Start all of these shoulder stretches and exercises with your spine erect and comfortably straight. Although I recommend doing these from a cross-legged position on the floor or a seated position in a chair for comfort and ease, there is no reason you can't do them standing as well.

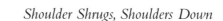

Shoulder Shrugs

Shoulder Shrugs, Shoulders Lifted

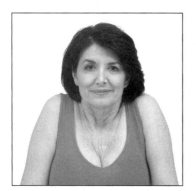

Shoulder Shrugs, Shoulders Lifted

As you inhale, slowly lift both shoulders up toward your ears.

Shoulder Shrugs, Shoulders Down

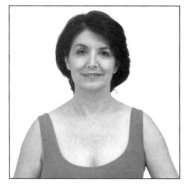

Shoulder Shrugs, Shoulders Down

As you exhale, lower your shoulders and press them down toward the floor.

Repeat 4 more times, for a total of 5 Shoulder Shrugs.

Shoulder Circles

As you inhale, lift your shoulders toward your ears.

Shoulders, Back/Shoulders, Down

As you exhale, roll your shoulders back and down.

Shoulders, Forward/Shoulders, Up

As you inhale, pull your shoulders forward and up.
   Make your circles as round as possible as you continue moving your shoulders back and down on your exhalation and forward and up on your inhalation.
   Do a total of 5 circles.
   Stop and change the direction of the movement.
   Inhale as you move your shoulders up and forward.
   Exhale as you roll them down and back.
   Continue for a total of 5 more shoulder circles.

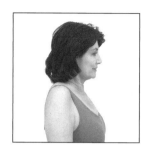

1. Shoulders, Back

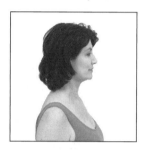

2. Shoulders, Down

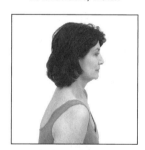

3. Shoulders, Forward

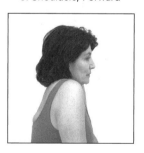

4. Shoulders, Up

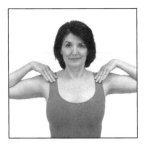

Elbows, Out to Sides

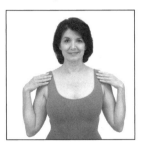

Elbows, Down

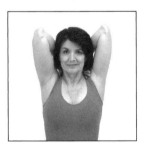

Elbows, Up

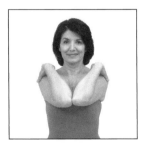

Elbows, Front and Together

Elbows in Four Directions

Elbows, Out to Sides

Place your fingertips on top of your shoulders.
   Lift your elbows straight out to your sides, shoulder high. Inhale.

Elbows, Down

Still touching your shoulders, lower your elbows and pull down as much as you can. Exhale.

Elbows, Up

Lift your elbows as high as you can. Inhale.

Elbows, Front and Together

Lower your elbows halfway, straight out to your sides, shoulder high. Bring your elbows to the front of you; touch them together if you can. Exhale.
   Move your elbows behind you as far as you can. Inhale.
   Return your elbows straight out to your sides, shoulder high, and repeat.

Elbow Circles

This movement is similar to the Shoulder Circles (see page 00), but the effects are different. Though your focus on these exercises will be on your elbows, the stretches benefit your shoulder muscles and joints.

Place your fingertips on top of your shoulders. As you inhale, raise your elbows up by your head. As you exhale, circle your elbows back and down. On the inhalation, bring them forward and up, and on the exhalation, circle them back and down. Continue for a total of 5.

Stop and change direction. Lift your elbows back and up as you breathe in. Move your elbows forward and down as you breathe out. Continue for a total of 5 more elbow circles.

Stop and release your hands to your lap while you take a deep breath in and out.

Namaste (NAH-MA-stay) is both a greeting that you will hear in the yoga world and the name of a mudra, a specific position for the hands. The stretch, Namaste Circles, refers to the placement of your hands held in prayer position at the heart. In a yoga class you will often hear the teacher say "Namaste" at the beginning or end of each class, addressing his/her students as the teacher brings his/her hands into the Namaste position. This is a way of greeting and honoring the class and means "the light in me and the greatest in me greets and honors the light in you and the greatest in you."

Namaste Circles

For the Namaste Circles, keep the palms of your hands together, and use the pressure of one palm against the other to create a circular motion in the space in front of you. The first set is a clockwise movement and the second set reverses the movement to counterclockwise.

If you are doing these from a chair, sit a little more forward in your chair.
Keep your back long and lifted without using the support of the back of the chair.
Your feet remain flat on the floor.

Namaste Circles, Palms Center

Bring your palms together in the center of your chest. Extend your elbows out to the sides.

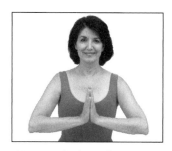

Namaste Circles, Palms Center

Namaste Circles, Palms Left

Use your right hand to push your left hand to the left and circle your hands in front of your chest.

Namaste Circles, Palms Above

Using a circular motion, raise your hands over your head.

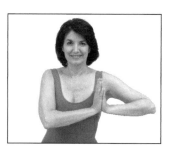

Namaste Circles, Palms Left

Namaste Circles, Palms Right

Bring your hands down to your right to complete the circle.

Next circle add the breathing. Inhale as you lift your hands (on the left side of the circle) and exhale as you lower your hands (on the right side of the circle).

Circle your palms for a total of 5 rotations.

Stop and reverse the direction of the circles for 5 more rotations.

Release your hands to your lap and sit quietly for a few moments.

Use the time to take an inventory of the sensations that the shoulder and arm stretches and exercises have created.

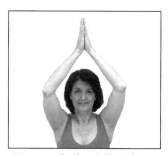

Namaste Circles, Palms Above

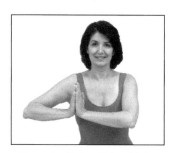

Namaste Circles, Palms Right

Like the rest of your body, your hands and fingers have joints and muscles that need attention to keep them supple and strong. You use your hands and fingers constantly throughout your waking hours, but you probably seldom think much about your hands unless they are in pain or are causing you trouble.

Stretching and flexing the muscles of your wrists and hands in these exercises will help to increase your hand strength as well as promote good circulation in your hands and wrists. The exercises also increase the mobility of your hands and fingers.

Hand and Wrist Exercises are especially beneficial if you use your hands in any repetitive movements for work or play. The exercises are therapeutic for repetitive strain injury and mild arthritis.

Whether you depend on strong hands or sit at a keyboard for your livelihood or you use your hands for activities like knitting or golf, add these easy-to-do stretches to your daily activities. They are convenient to fit in anywhere, while watching TV, sitting in traffic, or taking a break at work.

Make sure that you keep breathing while you do these hand exercises. Watch that you don't hold your breath as you concentrate. Aim for a deep, even rhythm to your breathing in each of the exercise segments.

Do these stretches and exercises for the wrists and hands from a cross-legged position on the floor or seated in a chair with your spine erect and comfortably straight if you are doing these as part of other Warm-ups or yoga poses. Extend your arms out in front of you, parallel to the floor, with your palms down.

If you are doing the exercises informally, adding them to your daily activities, you can do them from almost any position, for example, in your car, as mentioned previously.

Open and Close Hands

Closed Fists

Make two fists and squeeze them tight.

*Open and Close Hands, Fingers Wide Apart,
Palms Down*

Open your hands and spread your fingers wide.

Close back to a tight fist.
    Repeat 10 times in each position:
    Both palms face down.

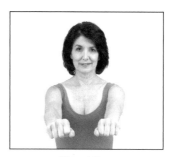

Closed Fists

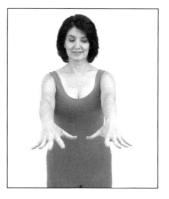

Open and Close Hands,
FingersWide Apart, Palms Down

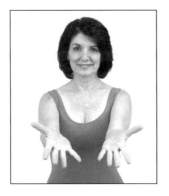

Open and Close Hands,
Fingers Wide Apart, Palms Up

Open and Close Hands, Fingers Wide Apart, Palms Up

Both palms face up.

Open and Close Hands, Palms Face Each Other

Palms facing one another.

Open and Close Hands, Hands Back to Back,
Palms Face Outward

Hands back-to-back, palms facing outward.

   Rest your hands in your lap and take a moment to feel the sensations in your hands as you sit quietly for the next several breaths in and out.

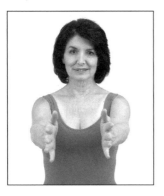

Open and Close Hands, Palms
Face Each Other

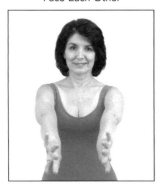

Hands Back-to-Back, Palms
Face Outward

Wrist Stretches

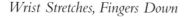

Wrist Stretches, Palms Facing Front, Fingers Up

Start the first two wrist stretches with your arms extended in front of you, wrists bent, fingers spread wide, and palms facing outward (the backs of your hands facing you). Move your fingers and hands in unison. Repeat each wrist movement ten times.

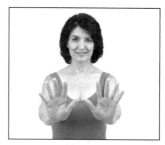

Wrist Stretches, Palms Facing Front, Fingers Up

Wrist Stretches, Fingers Down

Lower your fingers toward the floor, moving from the wrist.

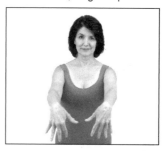

Wrist Stretches, Fingers Down

Wrist Stretches, Fingers Right

Lift your fingers and hands back up to the starting position.
   Rotate your hands to the left. This movement looks like windshield wipers on a car.

Wrist Stretches, Fingers Left

Rotate your hands to the left. This movement looks like windshield wipers on a car.
   Start the next exercise with your palms face down, fingers spread wide. This is the same windshield-wiper movement as above, with the palms facing the floor.
   Move your fingers toward the right, keeping your palms facing the floor.
   Move your fingers to the left.

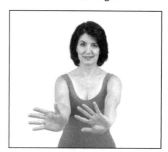

Wrist Stretches, Fingers Right

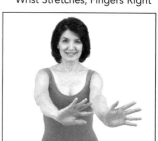

Wrist Stretches, Fingers Left

Rest your hands in your lap. Relax your arms and hands totally and be aware of the sensations in your hands and wrists.

•

Wrist Circles

With your arms extended in front of you, make two fists for these exercises. Move both fists at the same time. Rotate your fists 5 times in each direction.

Wrist Circles, Fists Turned in Toward Each Other

Slowly rotate your fists toward one another, circling each fist independently.

Wrist Circles, Fists Turned in the Same Direction

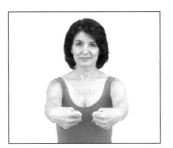

Wrist Circles, Fists Turned in
Toward Each Other

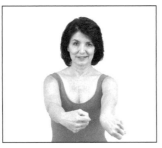

Wrist Circles, Fists Turned in the
Same Direction

Change the direction of the circles by rotating your fists away from each other.

Rotate your fists together in the same direction toward the right.

Change the direction of rotation of both fists toward the left.

Rest your hands in your lap and relax them while you take a few breaths.

Concentrate on the sensations that you identify in your hands, fingers, and wrists.

Few workout programs include the feet and ankles, but these exercises will be easy to learn and they are easy to do. Give your feet the extra care and attention they deserve.

These exercises stretch and strengthen the muscles around your ankles and in your feet, increase the flexibility and range of motion in your ankles, and increase circulation in your feet and toes.

One of my students swears by these ankle exercises. Recently, she misjudged the depth of a step and twisted her ankle as she stepped down. To her surprise she was able to recover her misstep with ease, and her ankle was not injured. She felt she was not hurt because doing these exercises had made her ankles strong and pliable.

Make sure to do these exercises with your shoes off so you can give your toes a good stretch. You can do them anywhere, and a great time is before you get out of bed in the morning or while you are seated at the edge of your bed.

There are no special breathing patterns to go with these foot exercises, so all you need to do is to keep breathing as you do them. Because there are no specific breathing instructions, this is where students in class have a tendency to hold their breath while they concentrate on the movements. I'll include breathing reminders so you won't forget to breathe.

Your position in your chair is the same for all these exercises: sit back in your chair and lift your legs out in front of you. Bring your legs parallel to the floor. This will work your leg muscles as well as your ankles and feet, so keep your legs straight and lifted throughout these stretches.

You can do these exercises while seated on the floor with your legs outstretched in front of you, although you get more of a workout for your legs when you do them from the chair position.

Ankle Flexes

Legs Extended, Ankles Flexed

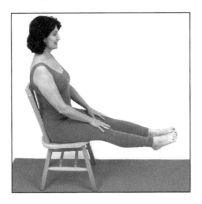

Legs Extended, Ankles Flexed

With your legs (lifted from the hips if you are in a chair) out in front of you, flex your ankles and bring your toes back toward you. Increase the stretch by pressing outward through your heels. Separate your toes, making as much space between them as you can.

Legs Extended, Toes Pointed

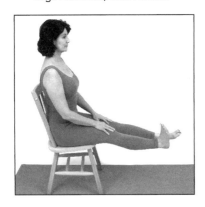

Legs Extended, Toes Pointed

Point your foot and toes away from you. Squeeze your toes together as you do this.

Repeat this Flex-and-Point movement 5 times. Are you breathing?

Relax your legs and lower your feet to the floor.

Rest your feet and ankles a moment as you take a deep breath in and out.

Legs Extended, One Ankle Flexed, the Other Pointed

Change the movement by flexing one foot while you point the other.

Alternate the position of each foot, moving both feet at the same time.

Do the Flex-and-Point movement 5 times (both feet).

Relax your legs and lower your feet to the floor.

Rest your feet a moment as you take a deep breath in and out.

Legs Extended, One Ankle Flexed, the Other Pointed

Ankle Circles

Lift your legs and keep them straight out in front of you. Move both feet at the same time. Start with your ankles flexed and rotate your ankles 5 times in each direction.

Legs Extended, Toes Out

Slowly rotate your feet away from one another, circling each foot independently.

Change the direction of the circles by rotating your feet toward each other.

Legs Extended, Feet Together to the Right

Rotate your feet together in the same direction toward the right.

Change the direction of rotation toward the left.

Relax your legs and lower your feet to the floor.

Rest your feet and take a deep breath in and out.

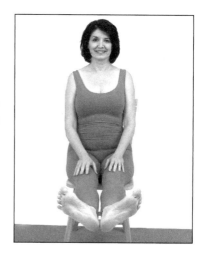

Legs Extended, Toes Out

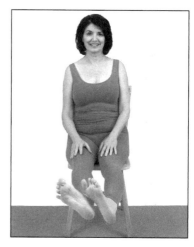

Legs Extended, Feet Together to the Right

Inward-and-Outward Ankle Rotation

CAUTION: Do not do this exercise if you have had a hip replacement.

Inward Rotation:

Lift your legs and keep them straight out in front of you.

Bring your toes together as you lift your outer heels. This is an inward rotation of the ankle and hip. Hold this position as you take a deep breath in and out.

Outward Rotation:

Bring your ankles together and turn your toes out. Lift your inner heels. This is an outward rotation of the ankle and hip. Hold this position as you take a deep breath in and out.

Alternate these two positions twice more.

Relax your legs and lower your feet to the floor.

Take a few deep breaths in and out while you focus your attention on the increased sensations in your feet and ankles.

Four

BASIC STANDING POSE

Thousands of tired, nerve-shaken, over-civilized people are beginning to find out that going to the mountain is going home.

—John Muir, (1838–1914) American naturalist and conservationist

MOUNTAIN POSE—TADASANA (TAH-DAHS-anna)

Mountain Pose looks so simple that an observer seeing you in Mountain Pose might think you are simply standing and doing nothing. However, as you experience Mountain Pose you will see that each part of your body is actively engaged. If Mountain Pose is new to you, your practice of it may seem awkward or stiff at first. With time, the pose will feel more natural, and your body will feel more open and expansive.

There is a mental aspect to Mountain Pose as well. You focus your gaze, observe your breathing, and bring your mind to the present instead of losing yourself in thoughts of the past or anticipation of the future.

Mountain Pose provides a solid foundation for the other standing poses because it is the basis for good postural alignment and is a means for centering yourself and developing concentration.

If you are unsure of your balance, practice this pose with a chair in front of you. Steady yourself by placing your fingertips on the back of the chair as you concentrate on the many fine adjustments you need to make to do the pose. Once you are in place, experiment with removing your hands from the chair. If you can take your arms to your sides, moving them out from your body a little may help in balancing. Tighten the muscles of your arms and extend your fingers. Don't forget to breathe as you are concentrating.

A good Mountain Pose is achieved through a series of specific postural adjustments starting with your feet. Your feet are the foundation of any standing pose, and you make your adjustments from the base up.

●

Feet

Stand barefoot so that you will be able to sense the bottoms of your feet and see your toes.

Place your feet a distance of 6 to 8 inches apart. Some schools of yoga suggest that the feet be placed together with the big toes touching for Mountain Pose. I prefer for you to stand with a wider stance so that your feet are right underneath your hips. This gives you a more stable base.

Bring your attention to the bottom of your feet. How are you standing? You often stand with more of your weight over one foot than the other. In Mountain Pose it is important to stand with your weight equally distributed. To sense this, experiment by moving your weight from side to side, first with more over the left foot and then with more over the right. Go from side to side several times. Stop when you feel your body weight evenly distributed over both feet.

Look down at your toes. After being confined in shoes for most of the day, toes are often cramped and look squeezed together. Are your toes scrunched together?

Press your weight down into the balls of your feet and lift all 10 toes up off the floor. Spread your toes as far apart as you can. Maintain this spacing and place your toes back down on the floor.

Balance your body weight so that it is evenly distributed over your toes and heels. You may need to shift your body weight from toes to heels a few times to note the difference in weight distribution and end balanced equally.

Press downward strongly and evenly into your toes, the balls of your feet, and your heels.

●

Legs

Contract your thigh muscles, which lift the kneecaps and help to stabilize your knees. Don't press or force your knees back, overstretching the backside of your knees.

Feel the upward pull of your leg muscles in contrast to the downward pressure of your feet. Imagine that your leg muscles "hug" the bones of your legs and that your legs are strong and long.

●

Hips and Spine

Gently move your pelvis directly over your ankles as you contract and pull in your abdominal muscles. If you have trouble finding your abdominal muscles, locate them by taking a belly breath. Relax your abdominal area outward on an inhalation and pull your lower belly in as you exhale.

Extend your spine upward, lifting and elongating the backbone.

●

Chest and Shoulders

Expand and broaden the front of your chest. Lift your sternum (the center bone where your ribs join together in the front of the chest).

Pull your shoulders back. Move your shoulder blades down your back and toward one another.

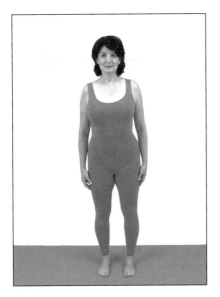

Mountain Pose

Don't lean back. Keep your shoulders directly above your hips.

●

Head

Let your head rest lightly on top of your spine. Fix your gaze on a spot directly in front of you and be aware of your breathing.

Your body should be aligned so that:

Your ears are in line with your shoulders,

Your shoulders are in line with your hips,

Your hips are in line with your ankles.

Locate that still place inside where you are steady as a mountain. Make your pose solid and still.

Keep your breathing even and regular. Hold the pose for up to a minute.

Mountain Pose

Go from Mountain Pose, to a relaxed standing posture, and back to Mountain Pose to become more familiar with the difference between your normal stance and this intentionally aligned posture.

> Try practicing Mountain Pose many times throughout your day, not just when you are doing yoga. Try it as you are waiting in line or standing in an elevator or on an escalator. See how experiencing Mountain Pose in new surroundings enables you to bring a moment of self-awareness into wherever you are.

Extended Mountain Pose

Stand facing the back of your chair in Mountain Pose.

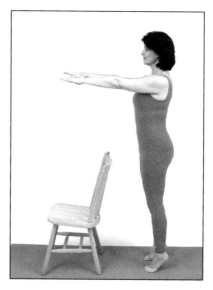

Extended Mountain Pose

Extended Mountain Pose

Place your hands on the back of the chair for balance and lift your heels high off the floor. As you move forward to balance on your toes, direct most of your weight over your big and second toes and draw your heels toward each other.

Keep your leg muscles strong and firm.

When you feel steady, raise your arms straight out in front of you, parallel to the floor, palms facing down. Make your arms strong and firm.

Balance on your toes with your heels lifted high and hold this position as long as you can.

Lower your heels and arms and return to Mountain Pose.

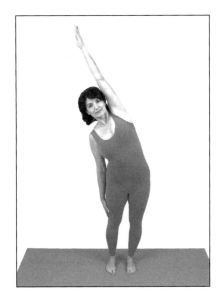

Mountain Pose Standing Side Stretch

Mountain Pose Standing Side Stretch

This is a great stretch for your torso. After doing it you will feel you can breathe easier and deeper and be more awake and invigorated. The stretch brings flexibility to the spine and tones the spinal muscles and nerves. It stretches the side of your body and the intercostals (muscles between the ribs) and helps bring definition to the waist.

Mountain Pose Standing Side Stretch

Stand in Mountain Pose, close to the back of your chair.

Place your right fingertips on the back of the chair.

To stretch to the right, extend your left arm above your head toward the ceiling. Reach up and feel the stretch through your left hand and arm.

Increase the stretch by raising your left shoulder and feel the stretch into your armpit area and down your left side to your hip. Let your ribs separate as you stretch the muscles between your ribs.

Inhale deeply. As you exhale, bend at the waist, sideways to the right.

Reach strongly through your left hand and arm, up and over your head to your right side in a diagonal line. Feel the space between your ribs opening even more.

Begin to breathe deeply. As you exhale each breath, take the stretch a little farther and deeper. Hold the stretch for at least three deep breaths or longer if you are comfortable.

To come out of the pose, inhale and lift your left arm and hand up toward the ceiling as you draw your torso back to an upright position.

Exhale and lower your left arm to your side.

YOGA FOR ALL OF US

Return to Mountain Pose.

Take a moment to observe the effects of the stretch before you move to do the other side. Does the left side of your chest feel more open, more awake and alive?

Repeat the stretch on the other side.

•

Mountain Pose Standing Side Stretch, Deeper

Adding movement of your hips will deepen the pose.

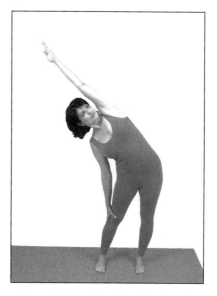

Mountain Pose Standing Side Stretch, Deeper and With Head Turned

Mountain Pose Standing Side Stretch, Deeper and with Head Turned

Come into the Standing Side Stretch to the right, your left arm extended up and over to the right.

Instead of keeping your weight centered evenly over both feet, push your left hip out to the left and shift most of your weight over your left foot to increase the stretch.

Keep your left arm straight. Actively reach up and over your head on a diagonal line.

Gently turn your head to look under your left arm, and gaze up at the ceiling.

Breathe deeply as before, holding the stretch for 3 breaths or more. On an inhalation, bring yourself upright.

Exhale as you lower your left arm to your side.

Return to Mountain Pose.

Repeat this deeper stretch to the other side.

When you are back in the Mountain Pose, note how your torso feels after completing the stretch for a second time on each side.

Five

STANDING BALANCE POSES

Refuse to let an old person move into your body.
—Wayne Dyer, author and motivational speaker

When seniors first start a yoga program, it is not uncommon to hear complaints that their balance has suffered or declined over the years. Many have become less sure of themselves when walking over uneven ground or on an irregular, unpaved surface. Using a stepladder may be out of the question, and some people experience difficulty and instability while standing on tiptoe to reach an object high in a topmost cupboard. Unfortunately, each one of us knows of someone who momentarily lost balance and fell, causing a fracture or break in a bone. Whether you are wobbly and afraid of losing your balance and falling, or you just don't want to get that way, you will benefit from regular practice of the standing balance poses.

Practice with a chair, which will add safety as you work on your ability to balance on one leg in these poses. There is no disadvantage to using the chair for support. Rather, the chair enables you to do the pose and gain its benefits without worry of falling. I have shown some of the standing balance poses without a chair so you can see the pose unobstructed. Please practice with the chair in place.

Place the chair so that the seat of the chair faces away from you. Stand to face the back of the chair.

Keep the fingers of one hand touching the back of the chair as you move into each pose.

Don't rush. Move slowly, both coming into a pose as well as out of it.

Hold your pose as still as possible. Then lightly lift your fingers off the chair to test your stability. If you don't feel steady, keep your fingers close to the chair back, if not right on it.

Focus your gaze on a stationary object in front of you. Not moving your eyes while in a balanced pose will keep you steadier.

There are many factors that can affect your sense of balance—from the muscles and nerves, to the inner ear, or the brain itself. Occasionally I have students who do not seem to improve their ability to hold balance poses unassisted for long, so they continue to use the chair. If your balance doesn't improve much, perhaps regular practice of these standing balance poses will help you keep it from getting worse.

I have heard many stories of how yoga has improved a student's quality of life in some small way. The following is a favorite of mine. A woman in her seventies confided to me that several months before she started coming to yoga class, she had had to give up taking baths. Her bathtub had no grip bars that she could use to steady herself, and she worried that she would lose her balance getting into or out of the tub. She switched to taking showers for safety's sake, but missed the luxury of soaking in a hot bath at the end of the day. Knowing that she needed to improve her balance, she practiced standing balance poses every day. It was only a matter of months before her confidence and surety returned, and she knew that she was steady enough to resume her evening soaks in the tub.

TREE POSE—*VRIKSASANA* (VRIK-SHAHS-anna)

Tree pose helps you build and maintain balance. The more you practice, the better your balance becomes. If Mountain Pose represents the ability to stand on your own two feet, imagine the accomplishment of standing on one foot!

Tree pose will strengthen the muscles of your ankles and legs, and will help increase flexibility in your hips and ankles, wrists and shoulders.

It is helpful to start learning this pose with a chair. If you know you can catch yourself if you lose your balance, you can practice without the fear of falling.

Bring a sense of fun and adventure as you practice the Tree Pose. That's how children approach this pose. They are not usually successful the first time they try standing on one leg, but they love to practice and they improve quickly. They don't get upset if they lose their balance; they laugh and try again. Be like a child when you practice Tree Pose. Have a sense of humor and smile!

> After taking my first yoga class, I discovered that I had been practicing a few yoga postures quite naturally. Tree Pose was one of them. As the oldest child in a large family, one of my chores was to do the dishes after the evening meal. It was not my favorite job; I was tired at the end of the day and didn't want to stand at the sink while others in my family could lounge or play. To amuse myself, I came up with the idea of standing on one leg, tucking my other foot up on my inner thigh. I turned the knee out to the side to fit against the sink counter. When the standing leg got tired, I switched to the other leg. Little did I know then that my practice of Tree Pose had begun. As a result, Tree Pose now feels so comfortable and familiar to my body that I can stand in the pose for long periods of time, quite balanced and at ease.

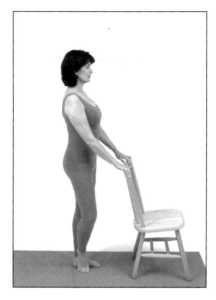

Tree Pose, Side View with Chair, Foot to Ankle, Hands to Chair

Find places to practice Tree Pose informally. For example, doing the dishes or as you are brushing your teeth in front of your bathroom sink in the morning and evening. Move your leg into position and hold onto the counter with your free hand. Make sure to practice the pose on each side.

Legs and Feet

Begin in Mountain Pose.

Tree Pose, Side View with Chair, Foot to Ankle, Hands to Chair

Shift your weight to your left leg. Look for the stability you feel in Mountain Pose on this one leg. Focus your gaze on one spot in front of you to aid in establishing your balance.

Keep your fingertips lightly touching the back of the chair as you pick up your right foot off the floor.

Turn your knee out to the side and bring the bottom of your right foot to the inside of your left leg. Place your right foot vertically along your standing leg, toes toward the floor, in one of three variations. They are presented in order of difficulty.

1. Put your heel above your ankle with your toes resting on the floor.

Tree Pose, Foot to Knee, Arms Out to Sides

2. Put your heel above your knee.

Tree Pose, Foot to Inner Thigh, Palms Together at Chest

3. Put your heel into your inner thigh, close to your groin. To move your foot up your leg this high you will need to use your hand to pull your foot into place.

Keep your hips level. If you have to lift your hip to keep your foot in the highest position, it's better to move your foot down your leg until your hips are level. Hip alignment is more important than where your foot rests on your standing leg.

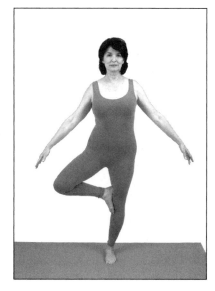

Tree Pose, Foot to Knee, Arms Out to Sides

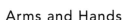

Arms and Hands

Continue to keep your gaze fixed on one spot to help you balance.

If you need the chair for balance, keep your left hand on the back of the chair and stretch your right arm above your head.

Make sure your hip does not rise up as you lift your hand over your head so you can keep the stretch along the side of your torso.

If you are balanced without the chair, you are free to move your arms into any one of these three arm variations. Try each of them; they are presented in or-

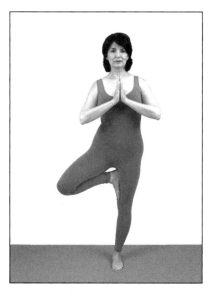

Tree Pose, Foot to Inner Thigh, Palms Together at Chest

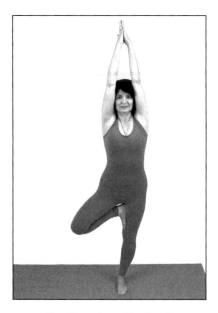

Tree Pose, Arms Overhead

der of difficulty:

1. Stretch your arms down and out to your sides, holding them a little ways out from your body (see photo top/page 69).
2. Press your palms together in front of your chest. Center your thumbs at your sternum and lift your elbows (see photo bottom/page 69).

Tree Pose, Arms Overhead

3. Stretch your arms up over your head and bring your palms together. Straighten your arms and lift your hands as high as possible toward the ceiling.

Return to Mountain Pose. Take a deep breath in and out. Repeat Tree Pose on the other side.

Remember to keep breathing as you hold the pose for as long as you can.

BALANCING WARRIOR POSE, WARRIOR III— VIRABHADRASANA III (VEER-AH-BAH-DRAHS-anna)

Of the three of the Warrior poses, Balancing Warrior Pose is the one that challenges you to improve your all-important balance. It firms and tones the area around your hips and the muscles of your buttocks and legs. Balancing Warrior Pose also helps you develop concentration, determination, and patience. When your arm position is in the overhead variation, you increase the strength, muscle tone, and flexibility of your arms and shoulders. Regular practice of the pose helps create better posture and builds stamina and endurance.

Balancing Warrior Pose is one that lends itself easily to being modified to be gentle and doable so you can practice it even if you don't have much strength or stamina. In its full and classical form, Balancing Warrior Pose is quite strenuous. With time and practice, you will be able to achieve the classical form.

Practice these variations of Balancing Warrior Pose before executing the full pose.

Balancing Warrior

Stand in Mountain Pose, facing the back of the chair and two steps away.

Beginning Balancing Warrior

Step forward fully onto your right foot, taking your weight off your left foot except for your left big toe, which touches the floor behind as you begin.

Contract your quadriceps (front thigh muscles), and keep the muscles in both legs firm. Keep your standing leg straight.

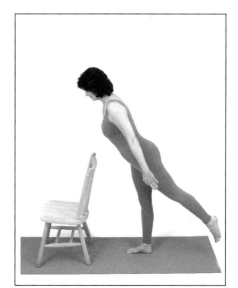

Beginning Balancing Warrior

Extend your arms down to your sides and a little away from your body to aid your balance. Use the chair if you need to steady yourself by placing your fingertips lightly on the back of the chair.

Lift your left leg behind you, just a few inches off the floor and as you do so, tilt your torso forward slightly. Keep your torso and back leg in line. Don't bend at the waist.

Hold the pose for several breaths in and out.

Lower your leg and step back to Mountain Pose.

If you are out of breath, even slightly, you need to breathe more deeply while you hold the pose. Remember to breathe as you move to the other leg.

Repeat the pose on the other leg.

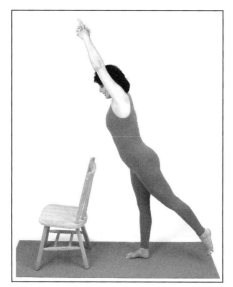

Beginning Balancing Warrior, Arms Extended Overhead

Beginning Balancing Warrior, Arms Extended Overhead

If you are not using the chair to steady yourself, try this variation with your arms. (This is a traditional position for the arms; many students say that the pose is easier to do using the arms this way because you stretch intensely from your fingers all the way to your toes.)

Beginning Balancing Warrior, Arms Extended Overhead

Before you lift your back leg, bring your arms into position. Lift your arms up over your head. Bring

YOGA FOR ALL OF US

your palms together, cross your thumbs, and stretch your fingers to the ceiling.

Straighten your arms if possible so that your upper arms touch your ears.

Keep your arms in line with your torso and leg as you do the pose. Return to Mountain Pose and repeat the pose on the other leg.

●

Supported Balancing Warrior

Take hold of the back of the chair with both hands. Step forward with your right leg.

Supported Balancing Warrior, Facing Back of the Chair

As you hold onto the chair, bend forward from your right (standing leg) hip.

Lower your torso as you lift your left leg up behind you so they move as one, bringing both torso and back leg parallel to the floor.

From the side, you have created a T shape. Depending on the size of your chair, you may be able to slide your hands from the back of the chair to the seat. Or turn the chair around if the back of your chair is in the way of your torso's forward bend

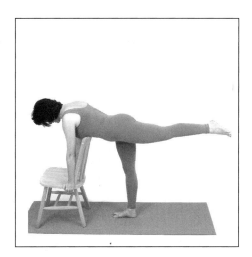

Supported Balancing Warrior, Facing
Back of the Chair

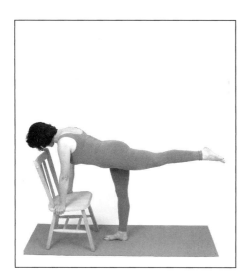

Supported Balancing Warrior, Facing
the Seat of the Chair

Supported Balancing Warrior, Facing the Seat of the Chair

Extend your toes out and away from your leg, and extend your spine and the top of your head out in the opposite direction. Feel as if you are stretching both your foot and your head out from the center of you.

Keep your standing leg straight, muscles firm and strong.

To come up, push yourself away from the chair and into an upright position.

Repeat on the other side, using the chair for support.

Balancing Warrior Pose, Warrior III

From Mountain Pose, choose an arm position that you tried previously:

1. Fingers touching the chair back for light support
2. Arms out from your sides
3. Arms overhead

Resume practice of the pose as in the previous version.

Balancing Warrior, Kwame in Full Pose

Lift your back leg as you lower your head and torso forward, keeping leg and torso in one straight line. If you can pivot forward only two or three inches, that's OK. Keep practicing and soon it will be ten inches and more. When possible, bring your leg and torso parallel to the floor, forming a T position with your body.

Extend energy out through your arms and fingers, spine and head, foot and toes.

Remember to breathe as you hold the Balancing Warrior Pose.

To help your balance once you are in position, keep your gaze focused on one spot in front of you.

Hold the pose for as long as you can.

Return to Mountain Pose.

Repeat the pose on the other leg.

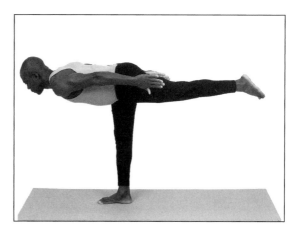

Balancing Warrior, Kwame in Full Pose

DANCER POSE—*NATARAJASANA*
(*NAH-TAH-RAH-JAS-ANNA*)

This is a lovely pose. Even in the beginning stages, you'll feel like a dancer.

Dancer Pose firms the muscles of your arms and legs, abdomen and buttocks, opens the heart and lung areas of your chest, and tones your spinal nerves and muscles, improving the strength and flexibility of your spine. And it works on balance and concentration. Because it gives a deep stretch to the muscles in the front of your thigh, Dancer Pose is a good counter to Warrior Poses I and II (see Standing Strength Poses, chapter 6), poses that build strength and power in your thighs.

Start with a Standing Knee-to-Chest Pose to help stretch the back of your thigh and your lower back in preparation for Dancer Pose. Without this stretch, the back of the thigh can sometimes cramp as you move into Dancer Pose.

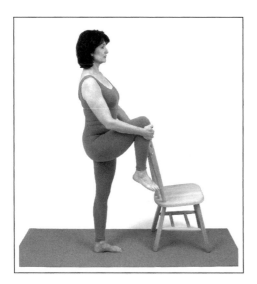

Standing Knee-to-Chest Stretch

CAUTION: If you have a knee replacement, do not bend your knee more than 90 degrees.

●

Standing Knee-to-Chest Pose

Stand facing the back of your chair.

Knee-to-Chest

Place your left hand on the chair back and turn your body slightly to the right so the chair won't be in your way.

Shift your weight to your left leg and foot and

raise your right knee.

Hug the knee to your chest with your right hand. You can hold on to your raised leg either in front of or behind your knee.

Test your balance and see if you can safely release your hand from the chair back.

If so, bring it to clasp your knee.

Hold for several breaths.

Return your left hand to the chair back.

Continue directly to Dancer Pose.

●

Dancer Pose

Dancer Pose, Preparation

Slide your right hand down your lower leg and take hold of the outside of your ankle. If you can't reach your ankle and you are wearing long

pants or leggings, take hold of the bottom of your leggings or pant leg. (If that doesn't work, move around to the side of your chair so that you can rest your bent knee on the seat of the chair, foot in back of you. Do not proceed farther.)

Drop your knee down toward the floor with your foot behind you. This is the position that gives an intense stretch to the front of your thigh.

While continuing to hold your ankle, thrust your foot backward and up while also pulling your foot as high as possible with your hand.

Don't let your knee move out to the side; keep it behind you.

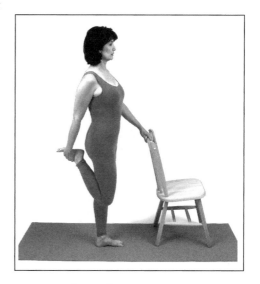

Dancer Pose, Preparation

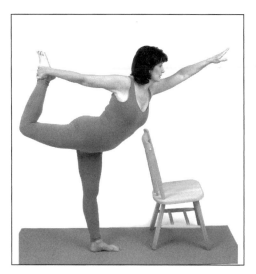

Dancer Pose, Full Pose

Dancer Pose, Full Pose

If your balance permits letting go of the chair, slowly remove your hand from the chair and extend your arm out in front of you, palm facing down. Raise your arm above shoulder height.

Let your torso move forward as your thigh lifts up behind you. Use the tension created by holding onto your foot to pull your right arm and shoulder back, stretching and opening your chest on that side.

Focus your gaze on one spot in front of you to aid balance and remember to keep breathing as you hold the pose for as long as you can.

Come into Mountain Pose and take a deep inhalation and exhalation.

Repeat the pose on the other leg beginning with the Standing Knee-to-Chest Stretch.

EAGLE POSE—GARUDASANA (GAH-ROO DAHS-anna)

This pose is named for *garuda*, a mythological being in India who is half-eagle and half-human. The *garuda* represents courage and one-pointed focus.

The compression and release of the entwining arms and legs in the Eagle Pose stimulate blood flow to these joints and also to the pelvic area. Flexibility is promoted in the ankles, knees, hips, shoulders, elbows, and wrists. This pose also relieves shoulder and neck tightness that contribute to tension headaches. The muscles of the arms, thighs, and calves are toned and strengthened.

The Eagle Pose improves balance, coordination, and concentration. Practice of the Eagle is a lesson in staying calm in the midst of constraint. This is a difficult pose, and part of your practice will be to remain centered while in it. One of yoga's extended benefits is the application of knowledge gained in the yoga poses to aspects of daily life. Eagle Pose teaches you to stay calm and focused during a challenging moment.

Some of your initial success with Eagle Pose will depend on your body proportion. This exotic-looking pose is more difficult for people with large biceps, heavy thighs, or short legs. Don't get discouraged if your arms or legs don't twist very well at first. Keep trying. The reality is that people who are thin have an easier time doing this pose. I know this from personal experience—the more I weigh (my weight has fluctuated over the past several decades), the more difficult it is to entwine my limbs in the pose. But whatever your weight or body proportion, I encourage you to do the best you can.

The following instructions isolate the lower and upper halves of your body position in the Eagle Pose so you can practice each separately before combining the two for the full pose. When you practice the Lower Body Position with the chair available, you needn't worry about balance as you stand on one leg and wrap your other leg around it. And because the arm position is tricky in this pose, practice the Upper Body Position before you try the full Eagle Pose while balanced on one leg.

CAUTION: Because of the twisting of the limbs, do not do this pose if you have had a joint replacement.

●

Eagle, Lower Body Position

Stand in Mountain Pose, your legs hip-width apart and the outer edges of your feet parallel to each other. This means that your toes turn in slightly.

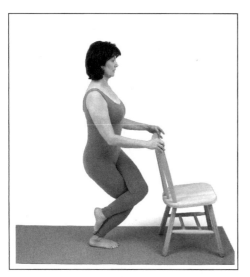

Eagle, Lower Body

Eagle, Lower Body

Bend both knees and shift your weight to over your right leg and foot.

Place your fingertips lightly on the back of the chair to steady yourself. Keep your back straight and your spine tall and extended.

Pick up your left leg as high as you can and cross it over your right thigh. Bring the outside of your left lower leg against the outside of your right lower leg.

Hook your left foot in back of your right ankle, so that your left leg is twisted around the right. If your left foot will not move around your right ankle, simply press your lower legs against one another.

If your hips have moved to the right while you've focused on your legs, center your hips to the back of the chair.

Keep your breathing smooth and even. Focus your gaze on a spot in front of you. If you feel stable, lift your hands from the chair and bring them out to your sides.

Hold this position as you take 3 slow, deep breaths in and out.

Return to Mountain Pose. Repeat the leg position on the other side.

●

Eagle, Upper Body Position

Start in Mountain Pose. Before engaging the arm position of Eagle Pose, bend both knees in Mountain Pose. Stay in this bent-knee position, your spine erect and tall. This will approximate the final stance without your having to balance on one leg. Keep your back straight and your chest open.

Eagle, Upper Body

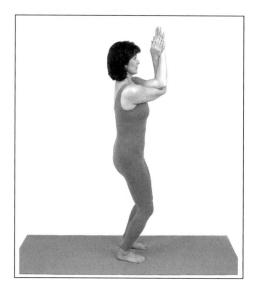

Bring both arms out from your sides, lifted shoulder high and parallel to the floor.

Lower your arms and cross your right arm underneath your left, bringing them in front of your body. (If you swing your arms down, you gain momentum for the next step.)

Bend your elbows and hook your right elbow under the left.

Raise your elbows to shoulder level, bringing your forearms together as much as possible. If you can, make one more half-twist and wrap your right hand around your left, bringing your palms together in front of you.

Eagle, Upper Body

Inhale deeply. As you exhale, pull down with your elbows and shoulders. Feel the stretch in the back of your shoulders. Hold for several breaths.

On an inhalation, lift your elbows as high as you can, keeping your lower arms perpendicular to the floor. Hold your arms in this stretch for several breaths.

Again, on an exhalation, pull your elbows and shoulders back down. Hold as you take several breaths.

Release your arms and bring them to your sides, and straighten your legs.

Return to Mountain Pose. Then practice the other side.

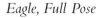

Eagle Pose

If you were able to lift your fingers from the back of the chair when you practiced the Lower Body Position, you are ready to combine Lower and Upper Body Positions. If not, practice each separately until you can safely put the two together for the full pose.

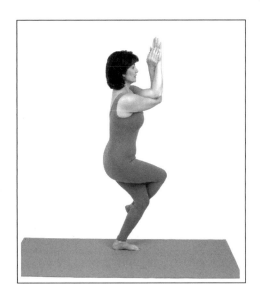

Eagle, Full Pose

Eagle, Full Pose

Move your legs into position first. Get balanced and steady, and only then add the arm position.

When the right leg is the standing leg, the right arm moves over the left.

Another way to think of the arm-leg coordination is that when the right leg moves over the left, the right arm moves under. However don't worry if you get the right/left mixed up because

YOGA FOR ALL OF US

different schools of yoga teach it differently. The way I teach it is the way I first learned the pose, but I have been taught both.

Focus your gaze as you hold the pose and remember to keep breathing.

Practice for as long as you can comfortably hold the pose—as little as 3 easy deep breaths to more than 10.

Return to Mountain Pose. Then repeat on the other side.

I have found an effective way to practice the leg portion of the Eagle Pose that will help coax your legs into position for the full pose. Do this while you are watching TV or are sitting at your desk.

Sit toward the front edge of your chair.

Cross your right leg over your left thigh.

Press your right lower leg against the outside of your left one.

Wrap your right foot around the back of your left ankle.

Keep the sole of your left foot on the floor, toes pointing straight ahead.

Hold for as long as is comfortable. Then release the wrap of your foot and leg and repeat the position on the other side.

Six

STANDING STRENGTH POSES

The most difficult yoga pose is that first step onto your mat.
—Judith Hanson Lasater, Ph.D., and physical therapist, Yoga teacher, author of *30 Essential Yoga Poses*

These standing poses are excellent for increasing muscle tone and leg strength, building stamina and endurance, and enhancing the mobility of your hip, knee, and ankle joints. They will aid in flexibility as well as promote better body alignment and symmetry.

If you have lost strength in your legs, regular practice of standing poses can help. As your thigh muscles grow stronger through doing these poses, you will find that you will be able to walk farther, climb stairs with greater ease, and feel more able and agile getting into and out of a vehicle.

As you practice these standing poses you will see your ability increase over time. The two most noticeable changes will be in the width of the stance that is comfortable for you in the standing poses (it will increase as you become more proficient) and the duration of time you can hold the pose.

In general, the wider your stance in the standing poses, the more difficult and challenging the pose is. As your leg muscles stretch and your hips become more flexible, you will be able to increase the distance between your feet. If your leg muscles and hips are tight, there is nothing wrong in starting with a narrow stance. "Start where you are and do what you can."

Over time you will also be able to remain in the poses longer and with greater ease. When a pose is new to you, it may feel like it takes tremendous energy to hold it for long. With practice the pose not only becomes easier to do, but actually becomes more invigorating and energizing.

I recommend that you perform each standing pose twice on each side. The first time, carefully position yourself and make sure your alignment is correct. Hold the pose for a short time, perhaps for only three breaths.

The second time you do the pose, try stretching a little farther than the first time. This time hold the pose for as long as possible while you remain relatively comfortable and steady, and come out of the pose as you tire.

Be sure to do each pose on both sides and hold both for the same amount of time. One way to determine the time is to count the number of deep and even breaths you take as you hold the position.

If you get out of breath, start to shake, or feel strain or pain, stop and return to Mountain Pose. Stay in Mountain Pose until your breathing has returned to normal and you feel your equilibrium return. Then continue where you left off, completing the second side or moving on to a new pose.

As my great aunt aged, she suffered a decline in leg strength and a gain in body weight. As she became less active, it became more difficult for her to get up and out of her favorite chair. One day she purchased a new chair, one that had a built-in mechanism to catapult her up and out. I remember as a kid being eager to try the chair myself, but it was hard for me to understand why Aunt Sue had so much difficulty getting up on her feet without it. As an able-bodied child, I thought standing up from sitting was simple. Of course what I didn't know then was that the less she used her leg muscles, the weaker they got, until the mechanical chair was a necessity. That chair and her struggles made quite an impression on me, one that inspires me to encourage my students to maintain or increase leg strength as they age.

POWERFUL POSE—UTKATASANA
(OOT-KAH-TAHS-ANNA)

Powerful Pose is sometimes called Chair Pose because it looks like you are just about to sit on a chair when you are in the pose. Powerful Pose is good for increasing the strength of your thighs, which is especially valuable if you have discovered that your quadriceps (front thigh muscles) have become weaker, for example, on that first day when you go skiing and your thighs burn or the time you have to climb many more stairs than you are used to and your legs become tired and shaky.

Powerful Pose also strengthens the muscles around your knees, ankles, and feet. It stretches your shoulders and chest and helps improve your posture. Powerful Pose is useful for tracking the progress of your endurance—the longer you can stay in position, the greater your endurance.

Powerful Pose is a warming pose when it's held for a half minute or more because the largest muscles in your body (thighs and buttocks) are active. The contraction of these big muscles creates heat, which circulates through your blood to your whole body and causes you to feel warmer.

Start with the preparation for Powerful Pose to make sure that your knees are properly aligned before proceeding into the full pose.

Powerful Pose, Preparation

Stand in Mountain Pose facing the back of your chair, with your feet about 6 inches apart and your toes turned slightly inward.

Rest your fingertips lightly on the chair back.

Keep your spine upright and your chest lifted as you bend your knees as far as you can without bending your torso forward.

Glance down to make sure that your knees bend right in line with your toes.

Do not permit your knees to splay out to the sides or fall in toward one another. It is important that your knees bend in the direction your toes are pointing. If your knees won't stay in line with your toes and the same distance apart as your feet, STOP. Bring your feet together with your big toes touching and your heels slightly separated. Perform the pose with your feet together and your knees together to eliminate strain on your knees. Done correctly this posture strengthens the muscles around your knees; done incorrectly, the muscles around your knees are subject to strain.

Powerful Pose, Preparation, Yoga Student Kwame

Once you have checked the alignment of your knees, move your head back to an upright position and gaze straight ahead.

If you are steady without the chair, move your arms a few inches out from your sides to test your balance. Make your arm and hand muscles firm by contracting the muscles, and press your shoulders downward as you lift the center of your chest.

If your balance remains steady, take your hands to your waist and draw your elbows behind you. This move stretches the muscles of your upper chest and helps to improve your posture.

Hold the pose; keep your gaze steady as you breathe in and out several times.

Return to Mountain Pose.

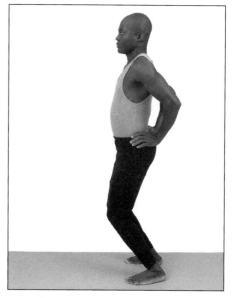

Powerful Pose, Preparation, Yoga Student Kwame

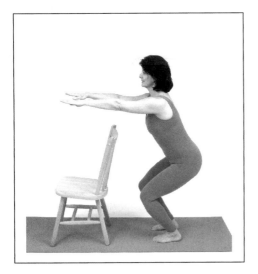

Powerful Pose, Arms Parallel to Floor

Powerful Pose

Powerful Pose, Arms Parallel to Floor

If you are steady without the support of the chair while in the Preparation above, resume that stance and extend your arms out in front of you, parallel to the floor.

Lean your torso forward and reach forward with your arms and hands as you bend your knees deeper.

Move your hips back as if you were about to sit on a chair but stopped moving before you were seated.

Keep your spine straight but inclined forward on a diagonal line.

Be sure to keep breathing as you hold this pose.

Return to Mountain Pose when you become tired or unsteady.

If you are out of breath, you need to breathe more quickly and forcefully as you hold Powerful Pose. Once you are in Mountain Pose, let your breathing return to normal before repeating the pose for a second time.

Powerful Pose, Raised Arms

Powerful Pose, Raised Arms, Yoga Student Kwame

Turn your palms to face each other as you keep your arms straight and parallel. Lift your arms overhead, reaching to the ceiling. The line of your arms continues the line of your torso.

Move your shoulders down away from your ears.

This arm position makes the pose more strenuous. If it is too difficult, lower your arms parallel to the floor, as described above.

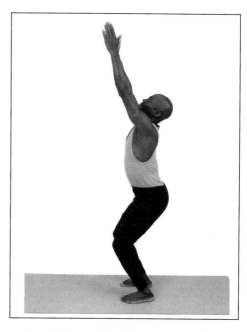

Powerful Pose, Raised Arms, Yoga Student Kwame

TRIANGLE POSE—TRIKONASANA
(TREE-KONE-AHS-ANNA)

Triangle Pose gets its name from the triangular shapes that are created in this pose. One triangle occurs within the legs and the floor, and another in the space outlined by the lower arm, leg, and side of the torso. Triangle Pose provides an intense stretch to the chest, hips, torso, legs, and internal organs. It increases flexibility in the joints of the feet, legs, hips, spine, and shoulders, and strengthens the muscles of the torso, neck, arms, legs, and ankles.

In the traditional Triangle Pose, you stand with your legs separated approximately 4 to 4½ feet. The wider your leg stance, the more your hips can move. But when you are first beginning to practice this pose, the traditional stance may feel too wide and be too much of a stretch for your inner thighs, so you may want to begin with a narrower stance.

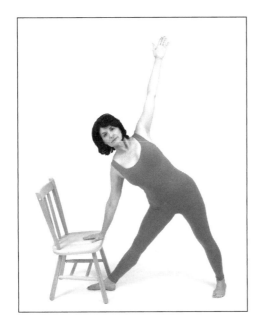

Triangle, Hand to the Chair

Triangle Pose

Triangle, Hand to the Chair

Stand with the seat of the chair to the right of you.

Separate your legs a minimum of 2 feet apart, and up to 4½ feet apart for the traditional stance.

Turn your right foot 90 degrees to the right, (pointing to the chair) and move your foot so that your heel aligns with the front legs of the chair.

Turn your left foot slightly to the right and press your left heel down into the floor.

Contract your leg muscles, making the muscles of both legs very firm.

Lift and extend your spine upward.

Place your hands on your hips.

Keep your back straight and tall and gently push your hips to the left as you lean to the right. Do not bend your spine. You may notice a tendency to curve your torso over to the right when you lean to the right, but do keep both sides of your torso straight and even.

With the chair: Rest your right hand on the seat of the chair and stretch your left hand toward the ceiling, fingers straight and extended upward.

Without the chair: Rest your right hand on your right knee and extend your left hand toward the ceiling, fingers straight and extended upward.

Don't let your left shoulder roll forward; keep it along the same plane as your right shoulder.

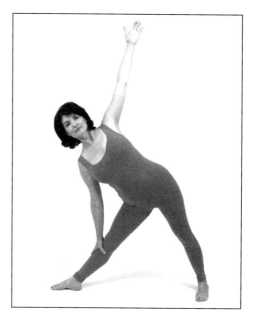

Triangle, Hand to Knee

Triangle, Hand to Knee

The wider your stance and the more open and flexible your hips, the farther down your leg you'll be able to move your right hand while still keeping your torso straight and long. In time your hand may reach to your ankle or to the floor beyond. Don't attempt to bend over farther than your flexibility presently allows because if you do push the stretch, you will either round the side of your torso or lean forward instead of staying over your hips. Proper alignment in Triangle Pose is more important than twisting your body to bring your torso and hand lower. The good news is that you get the full benefit of Triangle Pose wherever your right hand comes to rest. Initially, you may only be able to bend to the side a short distance. (With diligent practice, one day your torso will be a straight horizontal line from hip to shoulder and your arms a straight vertical line, right hand to left.)

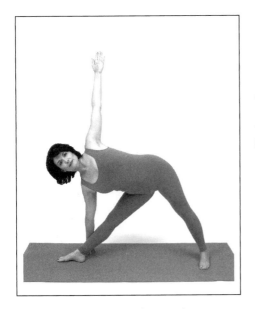

Triangle, Head Forward

Three Head Variations

Try all three to see which feels best for you. Avoid any position if you experience neck strain.

Triangle, Head Forward

1. Keep your head facing forward and your neck in line with the rest of your spine.

Triangle, Head Up

2. Turn your head to look up at your outstretched hand, focusing on your thumb.

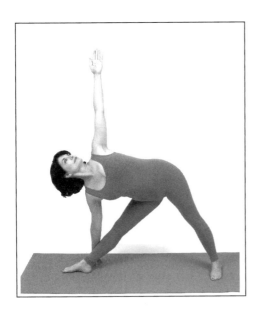

Triangle, Head Up

Triangle, Head Down

3. Turn your head to look down.

   With the chair: look at your hand resting on the chair.

   Without the chair: look at your right big toe.

Keep your breathing steady as you hold the pose for 5 breaths in and out.

To come out of the pose, lift your left hand up higher; and using the momentum of that lift, bring your torso up and lower your left arm.

Turn your right foot back to face the front, and move your legs together into Mountain Pose.

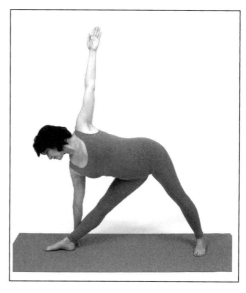

Triangle, Head Down

If you are using a chair for the pose, turn around to repeat the pose with your left side to the chair. Without a chair, you can remain facing in the same direction and turn your feet to the left to get into position.

Additional Hints

Press downward into your feet, and focus your awareness on your right big toe and your left heel. Pay attention to keeping the muscles of both legs fully engaged and firm. If you discover a tendency to let your right knee bend a little, resist and keep your leg very straight. As you press down into your feet, create a counterstretch up through your spine, elongating and lengthening your backbone.

Become aware of where you most feel the stretch in Triangle Pose. It may be your inner thigh or your hip, the side of your torso or your back, or even your ankle on the foot that is turned outward 90 degrees.

FRONT-FACING WARRIOR POSE, WARRIOR I— VIRABHADRASANA I (VEER-AH-BHAH-DRAHS-ANNA)

A fierce warrior in India, Virabhadra is this pose's namesake. He is the hero in an epic poem written in India during the fifth century. In Sanskrit, *vira* means "hero" and *bhadra* means "auspicious."

There are three well-known versions of the Warrior Pose, called I, II, and III, otherwise known as Front-Facing, Side-Facing, and Balancing Warrior. They all strengthen the legs and increase flexibility in the hips and groins. They stretch the calves and ankles, chest, shoulders and arms, and relieve stiffness in the upper back and neck. Each pose delivers the mental benefits of enhanced focus and concentration.

Warrior I and II are said to have positive psychological benefits in helping develop inner resources of courage and strength. Students have reported that these Warrior Poses feel empowering and a few say that regular practice of Warrior Poses have helped them feel internally stronger when they were going through tough and stressful times.

In their traditional forms, Warrior I and II are both practiced with the feet a distance of four to four and a half feet apart. Widespread legs make the poses quite challenging: your knee joint forms a 90-degree angle and your thigh comes parallel to the floor. The poses are less intense when you place your feet closer together than four feet. Find the distance where you can work to your full capacity without strain.

Warrior I is such a beneficial pose that it is one of the standards that I have my students do in class each week. I recommend that you, too, practice it often. In class I have each student use a chair as an aid for balance in getting into and out of this pose. Also, by placing your foot under the chair seat as you prepare for the pose, you prevent your knee from extending beyond your ankle when you are in Warrior I because the chair limits the forward movement of your bent knee.

Front-Facing Warrior I

Start in Mountain Pose, facing the back of your chair.

Front-Facing Warrior I, Preliminary Stretch, Legs Straight

Bring your fingertips to the chair to steady yourself as you move your legs into position.

Place your right foot underneath your chair, right heel in line with the back legs of the chair.

Step back with your left foot as far as you can reach. Place your left foot so that your toes turn out to the left enough to enable you to press your left heel down to the floor.

Contract the thigh muscles of both legs.

Move your hips to the right so that both your hips and shoulders face the chair.

Lift your hands from the chair back and place your hands on your hips. Draw your elbows behind you.

Balance in this stance with both legs straight.

Find a place of focus for your eyes and hold for a few breaths.

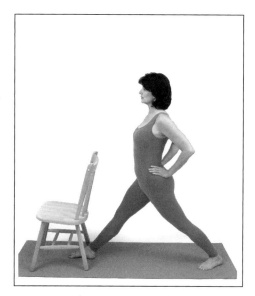

Front-Facing Warrior I, Preliminary Stretch, Legs Straight

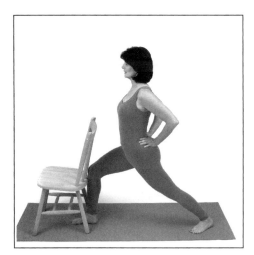

Front-Facing Warrior I, Hands to Hips

Front-Facing Warrior I, Hands to Hips

Return your fingers to the chair and bend your front leg until your bent knee lightly touches your chair seat. Keep your back leg completely straight.

Remove your hands and test your balance. If you are steady, take your hands to your hips and draw your elbows behind you. Push down against your hips as you lift your spine.

Look up. Find a place of focus for your eyes.

Imagine the sensation of stretching your torso in two opposing directions—upwards from the waist up and downward from the waist down.

Hold for 5 deep breaths or longer.

To come out of the pose, hold on to the back of the chair if you need to steady yourself and straighten your front knee. Step your back foot forward.

Come into Mountain Pose. Repeat on the other side.

Front-Facing Warrior I, Arms Overhead, Fingers Interlaced

When your front knee is bent, your back leg straight, and your balance steady, lift both arms overhead.

Bring your palms together.

Interlace your fingers and extend your index fingers upward, pointing to the ceiling.

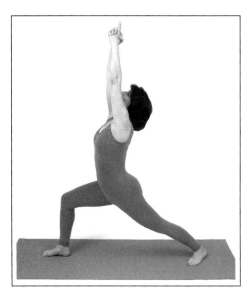

Front-Facing Warrior I, Arms Overhead, Fingers Interlaced

YOGA FOR ALL OF US

If it is uncomfortable to interlace your fingers, keep your arms straight, overhead and parallel, with palms facing.

Look up, lifting your chest as well.

Stretch upward from the waist as you sink down farther onto your bent leg.

The time you hold the pose is determined by your stamina.

To come out of the pose, slowly release your hands if you have interlaced your fingers, lower your arms, straighten your front knee, and step your back foot forward.

Return to Mountain Pose. Repeat on the other side.

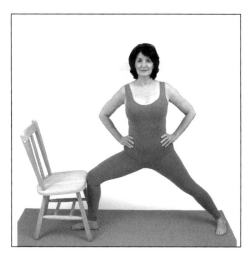

Side-Facing Warrior II, Hands to Hips

SIDE-FACING WARRIOR POSE, WARRIOR II—VIRABHADRASANA II (VEER-AH-BHAH-DRAHS-anna)

The second of the three Warrior poses, the Side-Facing Warrior, or Warrior II, has benefits similar to Warrior I: increased strength and flexibility in your legs, feet, hips, and back as well as stretch and toning for your chest and arms.

Also, as in Warrior I, when you practice Warrior II using a chair, the seat of the chair keeps your knee in a safe position by serving as a place marker for your bent knee, limiting its forward movement and preventing your knee from extending beyond your ankle.

•

Side-Facing Warrior II

Start in Mountain Pose, facing the seat of your chair.

Side-Facing Warrior II, Hands to Hips

Turn your body to the left so that the chair is to the right of you.

Separate your legs a minimum of 3 feet apart, and up to 4½ feet apart for the traditional stance.

Turn your right foot 90 degrees to the right (pointing to the chair) and place your foot so that your heel aligns with the legs of the chair.

Turn your left foot slightly to the right and press your left heel down into the floor.

Place your hands on your hips.

Extend and lengthen your spine upward.

Bend your right knee until it touches the chair seat, which brings your knee directly over your ankle. Keep your left leg completely straight.

Keep your spine perpendicular to the floor; don't lean toward your bent knee.

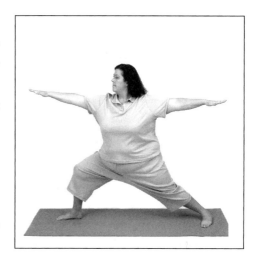

Side-Facing Warrior II, Arms Extended, Yoga Student Cathie

Extend your arms out from your sides, parallel to the floor with your palms down.

Turn your head to the right to look out past the fingers of your right hand. Find a point of focus for your gaze.

Side-Facing Warrior II, Arms Extended, Yoga Student Cathie

Be aware of your breathing and keep your breath steady and regular. With each exhalation, increase your concentration. Hold the pose for 5 full breaths or longer, as your stamina dictates.

To come out of the pose, straighten your right leg, lower your arms to your sides, and turn to face the chair seat.

Return to Mountain Pose. If your respiration or heartbeat has increased while practicing Warrior II, wait to practice the other side until both breathing and heartbeat are back to normal.

Repeat the pose on the other side, holding it for the same length of time as the first.

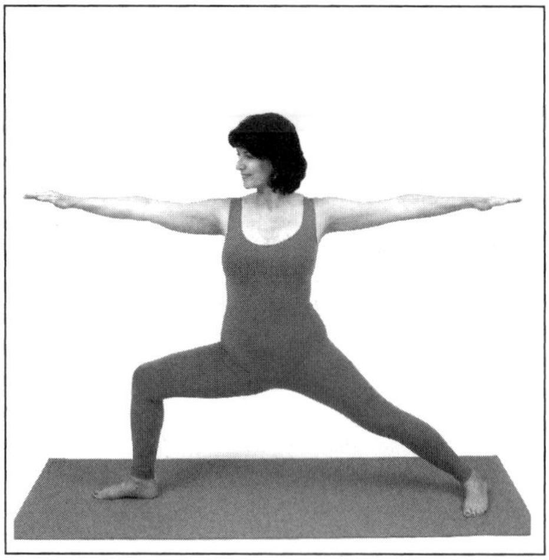

Side-Facing Warrior II

EXTENDED SIDE-ANGLE POSE— PARSVAKONASANA (PARSH-VAH-KOH-NAHS-anna)

Extended Side-Angle Pose gives an intense side stretch to the body, particularly at the hip, waist, and chest, underarms, and shoulders. It strengthens the legs and torso and increases the flexibility of the joints, especially the ankles, hips, and spine.

Practice this pose immediately after doing the Side-Facing Warrior Pose, Warrior II. Warrior II becomes the beginning position for the Extended Side-Angle Pose.

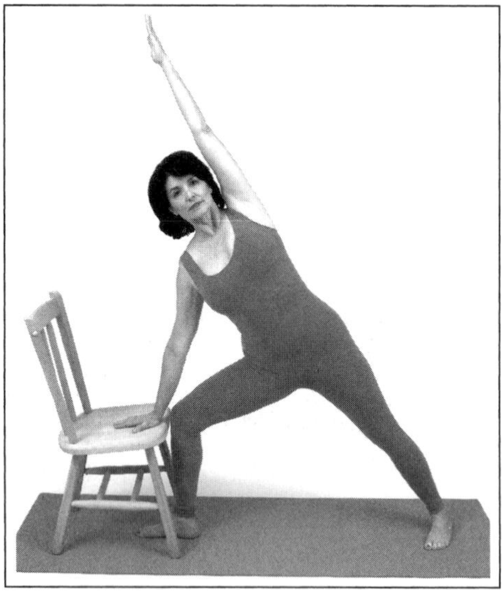

●

Extended Side-Angle Pose

Side-Facing Warrior II

Begin in Side-Facing Warrior Pose, Warrior II, on the right side. (See the instructions for the previous pose, page 101.)

Extended Side-Angle Pose, Hand to Chair

Reach to the right, leaning your torso into the stretch as you do.

With a chair: Drop your right hand to the chair seat. Take your left arm overhead, straight and close to your left ear. Turn your left hand palm face down.

Extended Side-Angle Pose, Hand to Chair

YOGA FOR ALL OF US

Keep your head inclined in line with your torso. Focus your eyes on a point in front of you.

Extended Side-Angle Pose, Elbow to Chair

If you can stretch more, place your right elbow on the seat of the chair.

Extended Side-Angle Pose, Elbow to Knee

If you are not using a chair, rest your right elbow on top of your right thigh by your knee. Take your left arm overhead, close to your left ear, keeping it straight and turning your palm down. Slowly turn your head to look up, underneath your arm. Focus your gaze up to the ceiling. Rotate your left ribs up and to the left to increase your stretch.

The goal is to create a long, diagonal line that extends from your left foot, up your left leg to your hip, through your torso and beyond into your left arm and hand.

Hold the pose as long as your stamina permits.

To come out of the pose, lower your left arm to your side as you straighten your right leg and come into an upright position with your torso.

Return to Mountain Pose. Then repeat the pose on the other side.

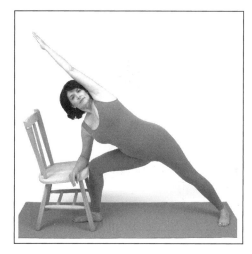

Extended Side-Angle Pose, Elbow to Chair

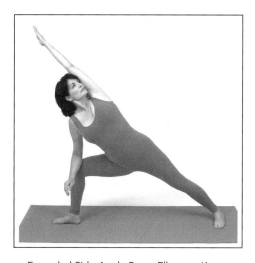

Extended Side-Angle Pose, Elbow to Knee

Seven

STANDING FORWARD BENDS

For fast-acting relief, try slowing down.
—Lily Tomlin, actress

Forward Bends are restful to mind and body and effective postures for releasing tightness in the lower back. In a Standing Forward Bend, the effect of gravity on the spine is reversed and places of compression in the spine are stretched and separated. Practice these poses if you experience strain or tension in your back after you have performed the Standing Balance Poses or the Standing Strength Poses because Forward Bends are a perfect counter to restore ease and comfort to your spine and the muscles of your back.

Forward Bends have a powerful and calming effect on the mind. When you bend your torso forward and your head becomes level with or lower than the trunk of your body, your nervous system quiets and your body and mind's natural inclination to look outward is reversed. In daily activity your senses are naturally tuned to pick up outside stimuli; when you bend your body forward in toward itself, your senses are directed inward. These Forward Bend Poses introduce you to your inner geography and give you an awareness of what is happening inside your body and mind.

When you are performing Standing Forward Bends, keep these points in mind:

As you bend forward, keep the spine long and extended. Don't allow the front of the torso to collapse or the back to round. Be careful to fold forward from your hip joints, not from your waist. To feel this action, stand tall and place your fingertips where your thigh bones join your torso and feel the movement as you bend forward from the hips.

Tight back and hamstring muscles will limit how far you can bend forward. To eliminate strain on tight muscles in your back or hamstrings, bend your knees slightly as you move into the Forward Bends.

CAUTION: If you know you have LOW blood pressure, come up very slowly from the Standing Forward Bends to give your body time to adjust to returning to an upright position. Coming up too quickly may cause you to feel dizzy.

CAUTION: If you have a back injury, spinal disc problems, or osteoporosis (low bone mass), check with your health care provider before practicing these postures. Avoid these poses if you are experiencing an acute sciatica problem.

> When I was invited to an elementary school to teach some yoga to the children, the teachers stayed to watch their students and observed the immediate effect of the first Forward Bend Pose. In anticipation of my visit, the third graders were active and rowdy. As soon as I entered the large classroom, I knew I needed to do something immediately to calm the children and to focus their attention on me and yoga. So I had them do a kneeling Forward Bend Pose called Child's Pose (Balasana), and I challenged them to stay in the pose for ten slow, deep breaths. After barely a minute, they sat up, transformed into quiet and interested children. Their astonished and appreciative teachers said to me after the class that they would be trying Child's Pose with their classes again.

This is a quick stretch, useful for relieving lower back tension. The beginning of this stretch is the same as that used to stretch the back of the leg before Dancer Pose, (see page 78).

CAUTION: If you have had a knee replacement, do not bend your knee more than 90 degrees.

●

Standing Knee-to-Chest Stretch

Stand facing the back of your chair.

Standing Knee-to-Chest Stretch, Hand to Knee

Place your left hand on the chair back and turn your body slightly to the right so the chair won't be in your way.

Shift your weight to your left leg and foot and raise your right knee.

Hug the knee to your chest with your right hand. You can hold on to your raised leg either in front of or behind your knee.

Hold for several breaths.

Pull against your knee or leg as you stretch your spine upward on an inhalation.

As you exhale, bend your head forward toward your knee.

As you inhale, lift your head and stretch your spine upward.

As you exhale, release your leg.

Come into Mountain Pose.

Repeat on the other side.

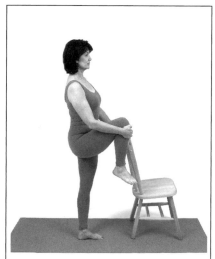

Standing Knee-to-Chest Stretch,
Hand to Knee

STANDING FORWARD BENDS

FORWARD BEND—Uttanasana (OO-TAN-AHS-anna)

The name of this pose really means "intense stretch" and if the backs of your legs are tight, it will feel intense as it is a strong forward-bending position. You can reduce some of the intensity by bending your knees slightly, which makes the pose more restful and comfortable.

●

Forward Bend, With a Chair

Stand in Mountain Pose facing the seat of your chair.

Forward Bend, Tight Hamstring Relief, Knees Bent, Yoga Student Ted

Bend forward from your hips, keeping your spine long and extended, and your back straight.

As you come forward, place your hands to the sides of the chair seat. Bring the top of your head to the seat of the chair. If you can't reach the chair seat, try bending your knees until the top of your head touches the chair. The pose becomes restorative and restful when you can rest your head on the chair.

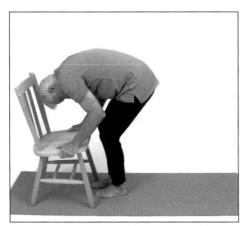

Forward Bend, Tight Hamstring Relief, Knees Bent, Yoga Student Ted

Forward Bend, Flexible Legs and Hips, Legs Straight

Instead of resting your head on the chair seat, hold onto the chair seat with extended arms (see also Downward-Facing Dog with a chair, page 114).

Stay in this position, aware of your breathing. Try counting to 10 breaths before coming up.

When you are ready to come up, bend your knees more and slowly uncurl your spine as you return to an upright position.

Keep your knees bent and your head tucked forward until you are all the way up. Return to Mountain Pose.

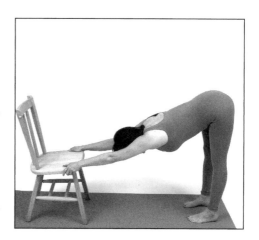

Forward Bend, Flexible Legs and Hips, Legs Straight

A "Less Intense" Forward Bend, with a Chair

You can obtain a gentler, yet very effective stretch by performing this pose facing the back of your chair. This is easy to do between Standing Poses and is especially helpful when you feel the need to stretch out tension in your lower back.

Forward Bend, from the Chair Back

Stand facing the back of your chair and hold onto the chair back.

Walk your feet back about 3 feet from the chair, bending forward as you do.

Drop your head down between your arms.

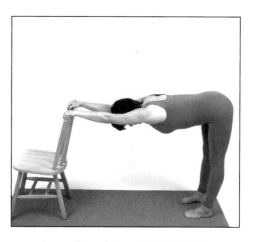

Forward Bend, from the Chair Back

Lengthen your spine, pushing your hips away from the chair. If your hamstrings (the muscles in the backs of your thighs) are tight and your spine rounds, bend your knees and lift your tailbone toward the ceiling to straighten and lengthen your spine.

Take several deep breaths.

To come out, lift your head and torso as you walk forward to the chair.

Return to Mountain Pose.

•

Forward Bend

To perform the pose without using a chair, start from Mountain Pose.

Bend forward from your hips, as far as possible.

If your hamstrings are tight, soften your knees by bending them as much as is comfortable.

Lift your tailbone toward the ceiling, slightly arching your back.

Choose one of three arm variations:

1. Let your arms hang from your shoulders.

Forward Bend, Hands to Elbows

2. Clasp each elbow with the opposite hand.

Forward Bend, Hands to Floor Beside Feet

3. Place your palms on the floor to the outsides of your feet.

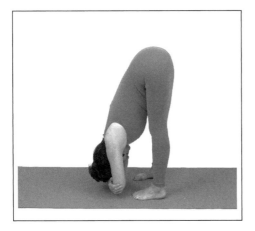

Forward Bend, Hands to Elbows

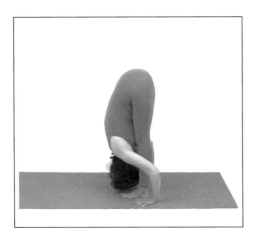

Forward Bend, Hands to Floor Beside Feet

YOGA FOR ALL OF US

Keep your neck and head loose. Let the force of gravity pull your spine downward.

Breathe slowly and evenly, and hold for as long as you are comfortable.

When you are ready to come up, bend your knees and keep them bent as you slowly roll up through your spine, letting your head come up last. When your head is all the way up, straighten your legs.

Return to Mountain Pose.

WIDE-LEGGED FORWARD BEND—PRASARITA PADOTTANASANA (PRA-SA-REE-TA PAH-DOH-TAN-AHS-ANNA)

This pose is a good release for a tight lower back or tension you may feel in your lower back after doing Standing Poses. The Wide-Leg Forward Bend is true to its name and the wider apart you can spread your legs, the easier the pose and more effective it will be. If your inner thighs are very tight, don't try to stretch them too far at first. Depending on your muscle tightness, there are two stances for the pose you can take.

Narrow: Use the width of your mat to determine the width of your stance. Stand on your mat and place your feet on the outer edges of your mat. Turn your toes in, keeping them on the mat and move your heels out and off the mat. Begin the pose from here.

Wide: Use the length of your mat. Stand on your mat lengthwise and spread your legs up to 4½ feet apart. Turn your toes in and your heels out.

●

Wide-Legged Forward Bend

Choose a stance from above.

Wide-Legged Forward Bend, Hands to Knees

Contract your leg muscles.

Place your hands on your hips. Bend forward from your hips, keeping your spine long and your back straight.

Slide your hands down your legs to your knees.

Stop there for a breath in and out.

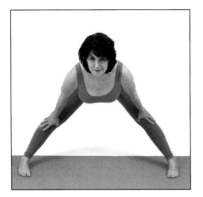

Wide-Legged Forward Bend, Hands to Knees

YOGA FOR ALL OF US

Wide-Legged Forward Bend, Hands to Ankles

Bend your torso farther forward and keep your head lowered as you slide your hands farther down your legs, to your ankles if possible.

Wide-Legged Forward Bend, Hands Between the Feet

If you can reach to your ankles with your legs in the wide stance, bend your elbows and place your hands between your feet. Move your elbows toward each other until your forearms are parallel.
Stay for several breaths up to a minute.

To come out of the pose, move your hands to your knees, and push against your knees to lift your torso halfway up. Then release your hands from your knees and bring yourself up to an upright position.

Walk your feet together and stand in Mountain Pose.

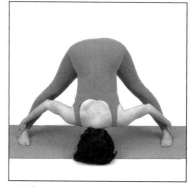

Wide-Legged Forward Bend, Hands to Ankles

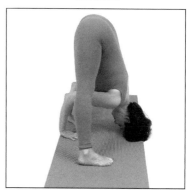

Wide-Legged Forward Bend, Hands Between the Feet

DOWNWARD-FACING DOG POSE—ADHO MUKHA SVANASANA (AH-DOH MOO-KAH SHVAH-NAHS-ANNA)

If you have a dog as a pet, you have seen a stretch very similar to Downward-Facing Dog Pose every time he wakes up. His pose stretches his whole body as this will yours. Downward-Facing Dog Pose makes the joints more flexible and strengthens muscles of the arms, legs, and torso.

CAUTION: If you have untreated HIGH blood pressure, skip this pose.

The first time you practice this pose, it may feel like it takes a lot of energy to hold it. Each time you return to it, especially after doing the Standing Strength Poses, it will actually become more restful and restorative.

·

Downward-Facing Dog Pose, with a Chair

Downward-Facing Dog Pose, Chair

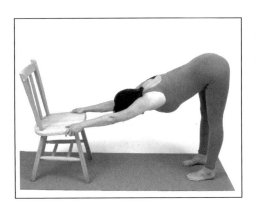

Downward-Facing Dog Pose, Chair

Stand in Mountain Pose facing the seat of your chair.

Come into Standing Forward Bend, holding onto the sides of the chair.

Step your feet back about 3 feet away from where your hands are on the seat of the chair.

Push away from your hands, straighten your arms, and bring your head down between your arms.

Make your spine long and straight.

YOGA FOR ALL OF US

If the backs of your legs are tight, bend your knees. While keeping your knees bent, lift your sitting bones up to the ceiling. This tilts the pelvis and helps create an arch in your lower back.

Hold the pose for 5 deep breaths in and out and longer as you increase your endurance.

To come out of the pose, walk your feet forward as you lift your head and torso.

Return to Mountain Pose.

●

Downward-Facing Dog Pose

Downward-Facing Dog, Table Pose, Hands Forward

Move to the floor and get down on your hands and knees, your hips over your knees, and your shoulders over your wrists in what is called Table Pose.

Walk your hands forward a handlength to create more distance between your hands and knees.

Spread your fingers wide, middle fingers pointing straight ahead. Press into your hands where your fingers join your palms.

Downward-Facing Dog, Knees Bent, Sitting Bones Lifted

Curl your toes under your feet and raise your knees from the floor.

Move your weight back onto your toes as you push away from your hands.

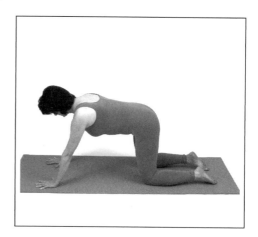

Downward-Facing Dog, Table Pose, Hands Forward

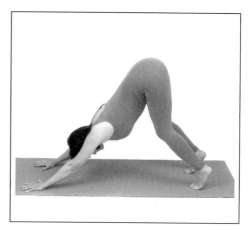

Downward-Facing Dog, Knees Bent, Sitting Bones Lifted

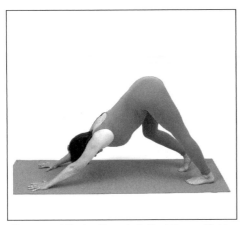

Downward-Facing Dog, Left Heel Down, Right
Heel Lifted

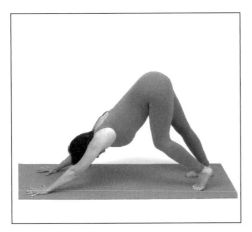

Downward-Facing Dog, Right Heel Down, Left
Heel Lifted

Contract and firm the muscles of your arms.
Keep your knees bent and lift your tailbone
toward the ceiling.

*Downward-Facing Dog, Left Heel Down, Right
Heel Lifted*

To help stretch the backs of your lower legs,
slowly straighten your left leg and press that
heel to the floor while you keep the opposite
knee bent.

*Downward-Facing Dog, Right Heel Down, Left
Heel Lifted*

Repeat on the other leg.
Alternate this movement to each side several
times, walking your feet in place.

YOGA FOR ALL OF US

Downward-Facing Dog, Full Pose, Legs Straight

Press both heels toward the floor and straighten both legs.

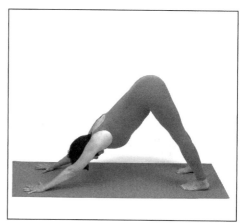

Downward-Facing Dog, Full Pose, Legs Straight

Don't worry if your heels don't reach the floor. It is difficult even for some yoga teachers to stretch their heels all the way to the floor with straight legs. If your back rounds when you straighten your legs, bend your knees again, lift your tailbone toward the ceiling, and push strongly away from your hands so that your spine becomes long and straight (see bottom-photo page 115).

Hold the pose for 5 deep breaths in and out, and longer as you increase your endurance.

To come out of the pose, drop your knees to the floor and return to Table Pose.

From here you can go into Child's Pose to stretch your back and rest.

CHILD'S POSE—BALASANA
(BAH-LAHS-anna)

This is a wonderful resting pose when done between other yoga postures, particularly after Downward-Facing Dog Pose. It gives a great stretch to the lower back and is calming to the mind.

Child's Pose does require flexibility in the ankles, knees, and hips to be comfortable. If you need to relieve some pressure on your knees while in Child's Pose, tightly roll up a towel and place it against the backs of your knees between your calves and thighs. You can also relieve pressure on your ankles by placing a rolled towel on the floor underneath your ankles.

CAUTION: Do not do Child's Pose if you have a serious knee injury, or have had a hip or knee replacement.

Child's Pose, Arms Extended

From your hands and knees on the floor (Table Pose, see top photo page 115), push your buttocks back to your heels.

Rest your head on the floor.
Two arm variations:

1. Stretch your arms out on the floor above your head as much as you can.

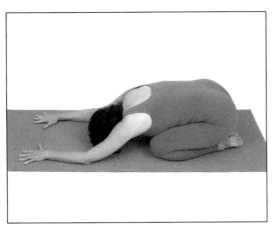

Child's Pose, Arms Extended

YOGA FOR ALL OF US

Child's Pose, Arms to Sides

2. Bring your arms to your sides, palms facing up to the sides of your feet.

Stay and rest in Child's Pose for as long as comfortable.

To come out of the pose:

From arm variation 1: Lift your hips and back to come to hands and knees.

From arm variation 2: Hold onto your heels and roll your spine up to an upright position. Return to Table Pose.

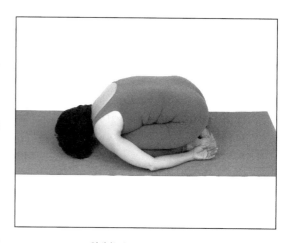

Child's Pose, Arms to Sides

Eight

RECLINING FLOOR STRETCHES

No one can get inner peace by pouncing on it.
—Harry Emerson Fosdick (1878–1969), professor, pastor, author

Stretches from a reclined position are very effective for your legs and back. If you spend much time sitting down, Western style (in a chair), it is common for the muscles in the backs of your legs to be tight. These muscles tighten also if you run, jog, or walk often.

When your hamstring muscles (those in the back of your thighs) are tight and inflexible, it is important to stretch them. Tight hamstrings pull excessively on the back muscles and contribute significantly to lower-back problems. If you have lower-back problems caused by muscle strain, start doing these stretches.

CAUTION: If your problems are disk related, be certain to check with your doctor for what exercises are safe for you.

When you lie down on your back, your back is supported by the floor and protected from strain. As your back rests on the floor, you can keep it straight without effort. In a supine position, your nervous system receives the message to relax, and the mind becomes quiet as well.

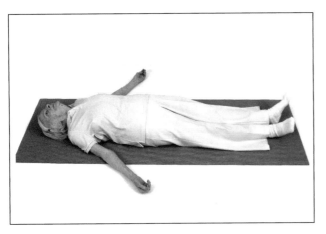

Reclining Floor Stretches, Chin Jutting Up

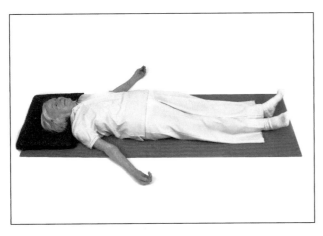

Reclining Floor Stretches, Face Level with Aid of a Folded Blanket

Reclining Floor Stretches, Chin Jutting Up

If your chin juts up toward the ceiling while you are in a reclining position, place a pillow or folded blanket underneath your head to bring your chin level with your forehead. This will help your neck relax and will feel more comfortable, too.

Yoga student Jo demonstrates most of the poses in this section.

Reclining Floor Stretches, Face Level with Aid of a Folded Blanket

These Reclining Stretches are a good and gentle way to begin a yoga session. Often I will start a yoga class with these to loosen the hips and stretch the legs before moving to the standing poses.

If you are very short on time and do only these poses, your body will thank you after even a few minutes of these Reclining Floor Stretches.

RECLINING KNEE-TO-CHEST POSE—PAVANMUKTASANA
(PA-WAN-MOOK-TAHS-ANNA)

In Sanskrit, this pose translates to "air freeing" or "wind-releasing pose." The position of the knee into the chest compresses the lower abdomen and helps remove gas trapped in the ascending and descending colon, thus relieving intestinal gas. The Knee-to-Chest Pose also increases hip flexibility and stretches the lower-back muscles.

•

Knee-to-Chest Pose

Lie on the floor on your back. Bend your knees and place your feet on the floor about hip-width apart.

Knee to Chest, Right Knee to Chest, Left Knee Bent

Lift your right foot off the floor. Bring your right knee toward your chest. Clasp your right knee and hug it into your chest. Keep your shoulders relaxed on the floor.

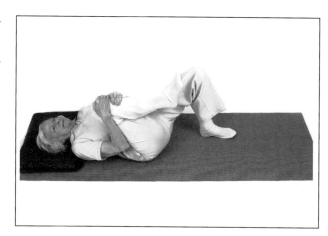

Knee to Chest, Right Knee to Chest, Left Knee Bent

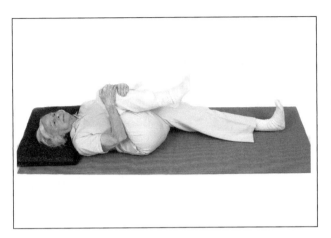

Knee to Chest, Right Knee to Chest, Left Leg Extended

Knee to Chest, Right Knee to Chest, Left Leg Extended

Continue to hold your right knee as you slowly slide and extend your left leg along the floor. Once your left leg is straight along the floor, flex your left ankle and press through your left heel. Press your left calf and thigh into the floor. Lower your chin toward your chest. Hold for several long, deep breaths.

Take a deep breath and on the next exhalation, lift your head off the floor and bring it to your knee, touching forehead to knee if possible.

Inhale and lower your head back to the floor. Release the hold of your right knee, and keeping the knee bent, bring your right foot to the floor. Bend your left knee and place your left foot on the floor next to the right, both knees bent.

Do each side twice, alternating from side to side.

YOGA FOR ALL OF US

Knee to Chest, Both Knees to Chest,
Head Lifted

Bring both knees into your chest. Wrap your arms around your knees and hug them tight.

Hold for several breaths.

Take a deep breath in and on your exhalation, lift your head to your knees.

Hold the position and breathe.

On an inhalation, lower your head to the floor and, with knees bent, lower your feet to the floor.

Straighten both legs along the floor.

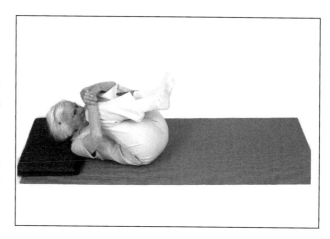

Knee to Chest, Both Knees to Chest, Head Lifted

Torso Stretch

Take your arms above your head and stretch your whole body. As you stretch, flex both ankles and press through your heels.

Increase the stretch more on the right side, reaching with your right hand and your right heel. Release the stretch.

Increase the stretch more on the left side, reaching with your left hand and your left heel.

Release the stretch.

Stretch both sides together evenly, reaching both hands and heels in opposite directions.

Release the stretch, bend both knees, and bring both feet to the floor.

RECLINING LEG STRETCH—SUPTA PADANGUSHTASANA
(SOUP-TAH POD-ANG-GOOSH-TAHS-ANNA)

The name of this pose in Sanskrit literally means "Lying Down-Foot-Big Toe Pose." If the hamstring muscles are stretched and loose, you can raise your leg while lying down, keep it straight, and reach up and take hold of your big toe. You may think that your arms are too short to ever be able to reach your foot this way, but your ability to reach your foot has to do with the tightness of the muscles in the back of your thigh and your hip flexibility rather than your arm length.

Regular practice of this pose stretches your hamstring and calf muscles, increases your hip flexibility, and tones all the muscles of your legs. This stretch is especially important if you have chronic lower-back tightness. When hamstring muscles are tight, they pull on the lower back and cause strain. Many people find backache relief through regularly stretching their hamstrings. Because you do this pose from a reclining position, your back is supported and stabilized while you work your legs. Make sure there is no strain on your neck; if your chin juts up toward the ceiling, put a pillow or folded blanket under your head.

·

Reclining Leg Stretch

Lie on your back.

Bend both knees and place both feet on the floor, about hip-width apart.

Hug your right knee into your chest. Keep your left foot on the floor.

Reclining Leg Stretch, Right Leg to Ceiling, Left Knee Bent

Straighten your right leg and stretch your right foot up to the ceiling. Clasp your right leg behind your thigh, knee, or calf, depending on how far you can comfortably reach.

Slowly flex your right ankle, bringing your toes toward your face, increasing the stretch in the back of your leg.

Gently, and with steady pressure, pull your right leg toward your head and torso.

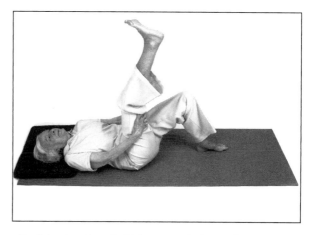

Reclining Leg Stretch, Right Leg to Ceiling, Left Knee Bent

Reclining Leg Stretch, Right Leg to Ceiling, Left Leg Straight

Once your right leg is extended, foot to ceiling, straighten your left leg along the floor. Press your left thigh against the floor, flex your left ankle, and push through your left heel. (If this is too intense a stretch for your legs, hips, or groin, return your left leg to the bent-knee position, left foot on the floor.)

Hold for up to 1 minute, breathing slowly and deeply.

To release the pose, bend your right knee and place your right foot on the floor.

Stretch out both legs along the floor.

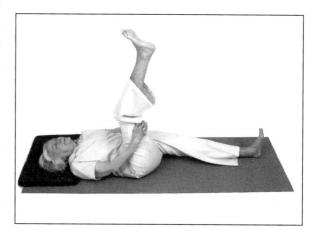

Reclining Leg Stretch, Right Leg to Ceiling, Left Leg Straight

Notice the immediate effects of the stretch. Some of my students say their right leg feels longer than their left (or vice versa), or that their right hip feels more open or is different from their left hip.

Repeat the stretch with your left leg.

●

Arm Extension

The use of a strap, belt, or towel acts as an arm extension to reach your foot. This is an alternative to holding the back of your leg in the Reclining Leg Stretch.

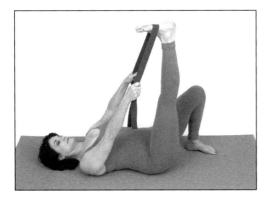

Reclining Leg Stretch, with an Arm Extension

Reclining Leg Stretch, with an Arm Extension

Place the strap around the bottom of your right foot and hold on to both sides of the strap before you extend your foot up to the ceiling.

Straighten your right leg.

Move your hands up the strap until your arms are straight. Don't bend your elbows.

Pull your leg toward you.

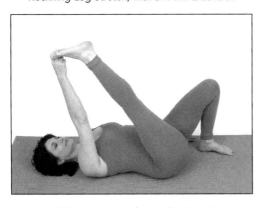

Reclining Leg Stretch, Hand to Big Toe

Reclining Leg Stretch, Hand to Big Toe

If you are able, reach up and clasp your foot or big toe instead of using the strap.

Gently pull your leg closer to your head and torso.

Keep your right leg straight and the thigh muscle firm. Don't bend your leg in order to draw it closer.

YOGA FOR ALL OF US

Tuck your chin slightly down toward your chest.

Hold the pose and breathe slowly and deeply for up to a minute.

Repeat the stretch with your left leg.

Reclining Leg Stretch, Both Legs Up

Repeat the instructions above, stretching both legs together as one.

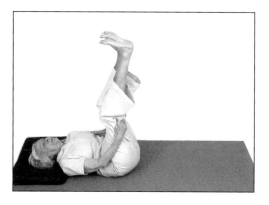

Reclining Leg Stretch, both Legs Up

Keep your hips and buttocks on the floor.

Hold for a minute keeping your breathing even and deep.

Release your legs, bend your knees, and hug them into your chest.

Stretch your legs out along the floor.

Then bend both knees again and place your feet on the floor.

Leg Cycles strengthen the abdominal muscles and muscles of the back, tone the abdominal organs, have a beneficial effect on the digestive system, and improve elimination. They also enhance coordinating breath and movement.

Begin as you have in the preceding floor exercises, lying down with your knees bent and your feet on the floor about hip–width apart. Press your lower back into the floor.

Leg Cycles

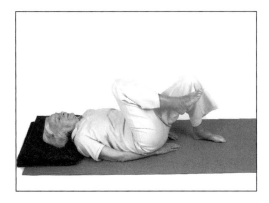

Reclining Leg Cycles, Knee to Chest

Reclining Leg Cycles, Knee to Chest

Bend your right knee into your chest. Place your hands, palms down underneath your buttocks to support your lower back.

Reclining Leg Cycles, Leg Straight to Ceiling

Straighten your right leg toward the ceiling.

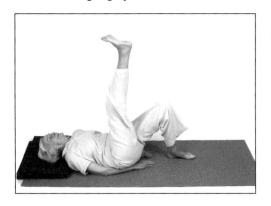

Reclining Leg Cycles, Leg Straight to Ceiling

Reclining Leg Cycles, Leg Lowered Then Extended, Parallel to Floor

On an exhalation, slowly lower the right leg toward the floor. Keep your right leg very straight, pull in your abdominal muscles, and press your lower back into the floor.

Lower your leg until you reach one of two points:

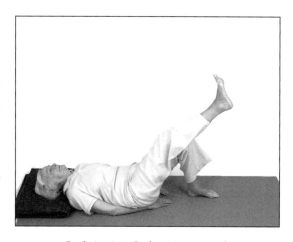

Reclining Leg Cycles, Leg Lowered

1. Whenever your lower back lifts off the floor.
2. When your leg is within a few inches of the floor (as long as you can keep your lower back pressed to the floor as your leg descends).

Then, as you breathe in, bend your right knee back into your chest. This is one complete cycle.

Repeat the cycle 5 times.

The breathing pattern that works well with this movement is as follows:

Inhale as you bend your knee into your chest and straighten your leg toward the ceiling.

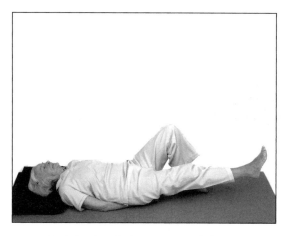

Reclining Leg Cycles, Leg Extended Long, Parallel to Floor

Exhale as you lower your leg toward the floor.

Reverse the cycle direction:

Lift your straight leg up to the ceiling as you inhale, and bend your knee into your chest.

As you exhale, straighten your leg outward in the air (to the place to where you were able to lower the leg when cycling in the previous direction).

Do not permit your lower back to come off the floor.

Cycle in this direction 5 times.

Rest with both legs straight on the floor and take a deep breath in and out.

Bend your knees, bring your feet to the floor, and repeat the cycles in both directions with the other leg.

RECLINING TWIST POSE—JATHARA PARIVARTANASANA
(JAH-TAR-ah PAR-ee-var-tan-AHS-anna)

Poses that twist the spine are an important addition to your yoga practice because Twists are a good remedy for the relief of minor backaches and tension held in the spine. I think of Twists as a way to give myself an easy spinal adjustment.

Twists stretch and strengthen the back and abdominal muscles, increase spinal mobility, stimulate the spinal nerves, and nourish the discs in the spinal column. Twists also gently massage the internal organs and, because of their revolving movement, help flush out toxins and wastes to be eliminated from the organs. Twists also stimulate elimination and aid intestinal function.

Reclining Twist Pose is helpful to neutralize the forward and backward movements of the spine from previous yoga poses.

CAUTION: If you have a serious lower back injury or are suffering from disc problems in your spine, do not practice these without the approval of your health care provider

●

Reclining Twist

Lie down on your back. Bring both knees into your chest.

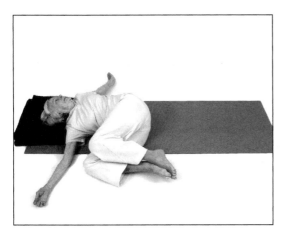

Reclining Twist, Right

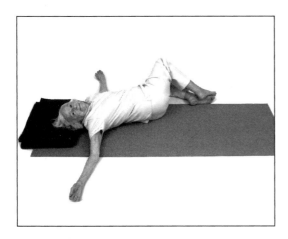

Reclining Twist, Left

Reclining Twist, Right

Open your arms out to either side forming a T with your torso.

On an exhalation, slowly lower your knees down to your right side.
Turn your head to look to the left, opposite to your knees.

Stretch through your left arm and shoulder and try to keep your left shoulder on the ground.

Once in the twist, place your right hand on top of your knees (which are lowered to your right) and apply a gentle downward pressure. If this feels helpful in deepening the twist, continue while you hold the pose.

As you hold the pose, keep your attention on your breathing and remain for 5 exhalations, or longer, as is comfortable.

On an inhalation, bring your knees back into your chest and your head back to your starting position.

Reclining Twist, Left

Repeat the movement this time lowering your knees to the left, for the pull through your right arm and shoulder.

Do two repetitions, alternating sides.

RECLINING HALF-BRIDGE POSE—SETU BANDHASANA
(SAY-TOO bhan-DAS-anna)

Half-Bridge Pose is a backward-bending pose that makes the spine more supple and flexible.

Backward bending of the spine is less common in daily activity than are the other spinal movements, but the spine needs to move backward as well as forward and side to side to remain fully mobile.

The Half-Bridge Pose strengthens your back, legs, abdomen, and hips. It stretches the front of your thighs and your chest, and tones your spinal nerves. The abdominal muscles and internal organs, particularly the colon and female reproductive organs, are stretched and massaged. The pose is useful for correcting rounded shoulders and is helpful in alleviating backaches. Holding the Half-Bridge for increasing lengths of time develops stamina and endurance.

CAUTION: Do not do this pose if you have a back or neck injury.

Half-Bridge Pose

Lie down on your back on the floor.

Reclining Half Bridge, Palms Down

If you have been using the support of a pillow or folded blanket underneath your head for the other reclining floor stretches, remove the blanket and set it aside.

Bend your knees and bring your feet to the floor. Place them as close to your buttocks as possible, and about hip-width apart.

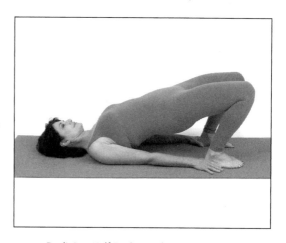

Reclining Half Bridge, Palms Down

Place your arms along the sides of your body, palms down.

Bring your attention to your breathing. On each of the next several exhalations, actively pull your abdominal muscles into your body. On the inhalations, soften your belly and let it rise on its own.

On an exhalation, press your feet and palms against the floor as you lift your tailbone off the floor.

Continue to lift your tailbone higher as you roll your spine up from the floor, first lifting your pelvis, then your lower, mid, and upper back.

Rest on your shoulder blades and shoulders.

Keep your thighs parallel to each other and your knees hip-width apart.

Hold for several deep, full breaths.

Slowly and smoothly, roll your spine back down to the floor.

When your back is on the floor, bend your knees and pull them into your chest. Lift your head to your knees.

Release your head and legs and straighten your legs on the floor.

Rest and relax for several breaths.

Repeat the pose a second time, holding it as long as your stamina allows. When you begin to tire in the pose, roll your spine back down to the floor, finishing as you did the first time.

Once your hips are lifted as high as is comfortable for you, you may want to move your arms into a position that gives additional support for holding the pose.

Reclining Half Bridge, Hands Clasped Underneath the Body

Move your arms underneath your body and clasp your hands together.

Straighten your arms, drawing your arms closer together.

Breathe slowly and deeply.

When you begin to tire in the pose, release the clasp of your hands and move your arms out from underneath your body. Then roll your spine back down to the floor.

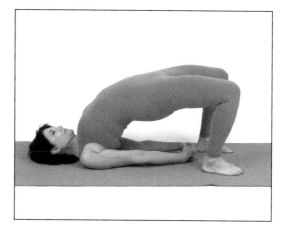

Reclining Half Bridge, Hands Clasped Underneath the Body

Reclining Half-Bridge Pose, Arms Overhead

Reclining Half Bridge, Arms on Floor Overhead

Before you move into the Half-Bridge Pose, lie on the floor and extend both arms along the floor overhead, palms facing up.

As you raise your hips and roll your back off the floor, your weight will transfer easily to your shoulders and arms.

When you begin to tire in the pose, slowly and smoothly roll your spine back down to the floor.

After your back is on the floor, lift your arms from the floor above you and bring them back to your sides.

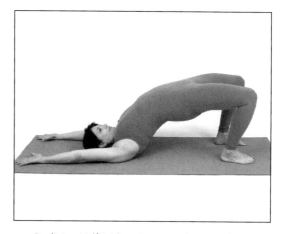

Reclining Half Bridge, Arms on Floor Overhead

RECLINING FLOOR STRETCHES

Nine

SEATED FLOOR POSES AND STRETCHES

We must learn to practice so that . . . (even) one minute of sitting will influence the rest of the day.
—Thich Nhat Hanh, Vietnamese monk and meditation teacher

The poses in this section are the most basic of the Seated Stretches. Practicing these poses and stretches will strengthen your back muscles, open and add flexibility to your hips, stretch your legs and inner thighs, and improve your posture.

As simple as these poses are, they may feel foreign to you if you are used to sitting only in chairs. I encourage you to try them daily. At first your back and hips may ache a little from practice; don't get discouraged—soon your back muscles will get stronger, and your hips will loosen and become more open. With regular practice you will see and feel improvement.

If tight hip joints cause your back to round when you are seated on the floor, place a firm pillow or a folded blanket underneath your buttocks to raise them. Sitting on the blanket helps drop your knees even with or lower than your pelvis to bring a natural (concave) curve into your lower back. If sitting upright using the folded blanket is still uncomfortable, you can sit with your back against a wall, or a firm piece of furniture, for extra support.

These are the postures you'll use for meditation practice (see chapter

12) unless you sit in a chair. When positioned properly, you'll find that once your body quiets in any of these poses, your mind will naturally quiet as well, even without meditating.

Yoga student Cathie demonstrates the poses in this chapter.

STAFF POSE—DANDASANA (DAHN-DAS-anna)

For several thousand years in India, instruction in Yoga has been handed down through an oral tradition from teacher to individual student. Yoga was not studied in classes or through books, and only a few ancient Yogic texts exist. The descriptions of the Yoga poses in them, unlike books of today, are simple and without elaboration. Staff Pose is described (in the *Yoga-Bhashya*) as: "One should sit down with the feet stretched out and close together" (Georg Feuerstein, *The Shamblala Encyclopedia of Yoga*), which is an accurate description.

However, as easy as the pose is, its physical benefits are plentiful. Staff Pose strengthens all of the back muscles and improves posture. It also helps to broaden the chest by stretching the muscles that run between the shoulders and the sternum (breastbone), which, when tight, are a contributing factor to poor posture. Additionally, this pose stretches the legs and tones the arms.

Staff Pose also works to discipline the mind and is a good seated posture for centering yourself and increasing your ability to focus. Staff Pose is a foundation pose for other seated poses much as Mountain Pose is the foundation for the standing poses.

Staff Pose

Sit on the floor and extend your legs out in front of you.

Staff Pose

Contract the muscles of your legs.
   Flex your ankles and bring your toes toward

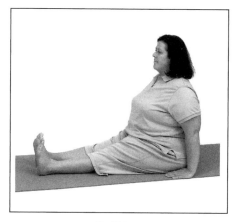

Staff Pose

you. While keeping your heels on the floor, press out through your heels.

Place your hands on the floor to the sides of your hips with your palms down and your fingers pointing toward your feet.

Press down on the floor and extend your spine and lift your sternum.

Pull your shoulders back and down, move your shoulder blades toward each other, and broaden your chest. Keep your chin level to the floor.

Create two imaginary lines of energy:

One running from your hips through your legs and out beyond your heels, and the other running up from the base of your spine and out through the top of your head.

Hold still in this pose for up to a minute while you breathe evenly. Remain aware of each breath in and out.

SEATED WIDE-LEG POSE—UPAVISTA KONASANA
(OO-PA-VEE-STAH CONE-AHS-ANNA)

This pose is the wide-leg complement to the Staff Pose. The Seated Wide-Leg Pose stretches the insides of the thighs as well as the backs of the legs. With regular practice in this pose, your legs will be able to separate farther and your hips will open and become more flexible, allowing you to bend forward with greater ease.

•

Seated Wide-Leg Pose

From Staff Pose, place your hands on the floor behind you and lean back on your hands. Separate your legs as wide as is comfortable.

Push away from your hands to an upright position and place your hands on your knees. If you can no longer keep your spine lifted and straight, stop here and return your hands to the floor behind you. Push away from your hands to lift your spine.

Flex your ankles and point your toes toward the ceiling. Press outward through your heels as you press your thighs to the floor.

Continue to lift and extend your spine upward.

If you can, bend forward from your hips and place your hands on the floor between your legs.

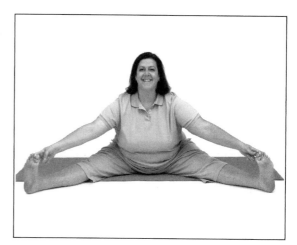

Seated Wide-Leg Pose, Hands to Toes

Seated Wide-Leg Pose, Hands to Toes

Walk your hands forward as far as possible. As you lean forward, take hold of your toes if you can reach them. If not, keep your hands on the floor in front of you.

Keep your toes pointing toward the ceiling. Don't let your knees roll inward.

Hold the pose for 10 deep breaths in and out.

Walk your hands back along the floor toward your body until your spine is upright and your torso is no longer leaning forward.

Bend your knees a little and, with the help of your hands, push your knees together.

Straighten your legs and return to Staff Pose.

CROSS-LEGGED POSE AND STRETCHES—SUKASANA
(su-KAHS-anna)

The literal translation of Sukasana is "easy pose." In ancient texts Cross-legged Pose is described as a posture "through which steadiness can be gained" (Georg Feuerstein, *The Shambhala Encyclopedia Of Yoga*). This is a recommended pose for the practice of meditation and is suggested for people who cannot sit in other more difficult seated poses like the well-known Full Lotus Pose, Padmasana (where, in a cross-legged position, the feet are crossed and the soles are turned upward and rest on top of the thighs).

The Cross-legged Pose is very beneficial for strengthening the muscles of the back and torso, creating flexibility in the ankles and loosening and opening the hips. Though it may take some time, with practice in this pose, your knees will move lower to the ground as your hips open.

I recommend sitting in a cross-legged pose every day for at least a couple of minutes. If your feet or legs fall asleep or are uncomfortable, you may need to start with only a minute or two in the pose and work your way up to more time. For every few days of practice, add a minute to the time you are in the pose, until you can go for five or ten minutes at a stretch.

Remember, it will be more comfortable to sit on a firm pillow or a couple of folded blankets to raise your hips higher than your knees; this support provides relief to your hips, knees, and ankle joints.

If you have mild pain in your knees when you sit in a cross-legged pose, try relieving any knee discomfort by placing a firmly rolled washcloth behind each knee before bending it.

CAUTION: If you have a knee injury, be most attentive to your knees and come out of the pose if your knee hurts.

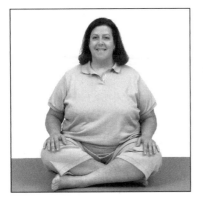

Cross-legged Pose

Cross-legged Pose

While sitting on the floor, bend your knees and cross your lower legs, bringing your right ankle underneath your left.

Rest your hands on your knees.

Cross-legged Pose

Sit tall and still.

After a minute of sitting, change the cross of your legs. Sit tall and still for another minute.

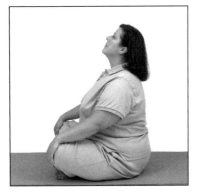

Cross-legged Pose, Side View, Extension Stretch

Cross-legged Pose, Extension Stretch

Once you are comfortably in the pose, place your hands around your knees.

Cross-legged Pose, Side View, Extension Stretch

As you inhale, stretch your spine upward, pull your shoulders back, and look up. Use your hands against your knees to get increased lift in your spine.

As you exhale, release the stretch of the spine and head.

Do this twice more.

Continue to sit in Cross-legged Pose, relaxed but not slumped, observing your breathing for a minute.

Change the cross of your legs and perform the spinal stretch again with three breaths.

Finish with an additional minute of relaxed sitting in Cross-legged Pose.

Cross-legged Pose, Forward-Bend Stretch

Sit as above in Cross-legged Pose. Take a deep breath in.

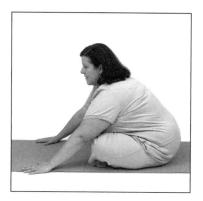

Cross-legged Pose, Forward-Bend Stretch

Cross-legged Pose, Forward-Bend Stretch

As you exhale, bend from your hips (not your waist) and lean forward.

Release your hands from your knees and place them on the floor in front of you.

Walk your hands away from you on the floor, allowing your back to round. Bring your head as close as possible to the floor, resting it on the floor if flexibility allows. Stay in this position for several breaths.

On an inhalation, slowly walk your hands back, uncurl your spine, and return to the upright Cross-legged Pose.

Change the cross of your legs as above, and repeat.

I had an older man enroll in my yoga classes for the sole purpose of gaining ease while sitting in the Cross-legged Pose. He wanted to learn how to meditate in this pose and be comfortable doing it. In the beginning his hips were extremely tight, and his knees were high off the floor. But he was determined to master this position. It took a year and a half of persistence! While that may sound like a discouraging amount of time, it did take awhile to make such a big change to years and years of stiffness; and in that time he not only acquired a beautiful and steady Cross-legged Pose with his knees fully open and wide, he also developed a welcome suppleness throughout his whole body.

BOUND-ANGLE POSE—BADDHAKONASANA
(BAH-DAH-KONE-AHS-anna)

The name "Bound-Angle Pose" is a literal translation of the Sanskrit. The pose is also called the Cobbler's Pose because it is a position used by shoemakers in India, who often work while seated on the ground. By holding the shoe with his feet, the shoemaker can use both hands to work on the shoe.

The Bound-Angle Pose strengthens the muscles of the back and torso, gives an intense stretch to the inner thighs and *groin* (the area between the tops of the thighs and the abdomen), increases blood flow to the groin area, and promotes health in the urinary and lower digestive systems as well as the reproductive organs, particularly the uterus in women.

CAUTION: Do not practice this pose if you have chronic knee pain or a knee injury. If you have had a knee or hip replacement, check with your doctor first and then modify the pose: once you have the soles of your feet together, keep your feet out from your body enough so that your knee joint forms no less than a 90-degree angle; do not pull your feet close to the groin.

Bound-Angle Pose

From the Staff Pose, bend your knees, open them to your sides, and bring the soles of your feet together.

Place your hands on your ankles or shins and gently pull your feet in toward the center of your body, as close as you can. You can keep your feet together or, alternatively, keep only the outer edges of your feet together and open the soles of your feet like a book.

If your lower back rounds in this position, remember that you will benefit by placing a firm pillow or folded blanket under your hips.

Bound-Angle Pose, Hands Behind

If it is difficult to sit up straight in this position, take your fingertips to the floor or the blanket behind you. Push your torso and pelvis forward, away from your fingers.

Bound-Angle Pose, Hands to Ankles

When you can sit comfortably without the use of your hands behind you, bring your hands to your ankles or shins.

Pull against your ankles or legs to elongate and lift your spine.

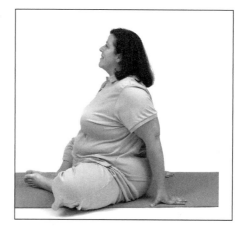

Bound-Angle Pose, Hands Behind

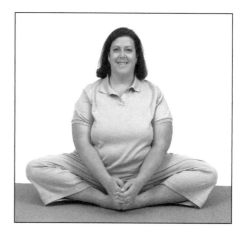

Bound-Angle Pose, Hands to Ankles

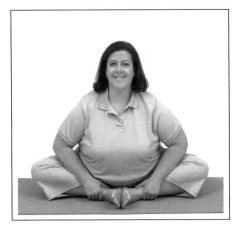

Bound-Angle Stretch, Elbows to Knees

Bound-Angle Stretch

From the above position:

Keep a long, tall spine, pull against your ankles, and bend forward from your hips.

Bound-Angle Stretch, Elbows to Knees

Place your elbows on your knees, press down, and gently push your knees closer to the floor. If you have a long torso, as I do, you may need to use your hands rather than your elbows to press your knees down toward the floor.

Be aware of your breathing as you hold the pose for up to a minute.

Return to an upright position, move your hands to your knees, and lift your knees up and together. Hug your knees into your chest, and then stretch out your legs in front of you.

Lightly massage your hips, knees, and ankles.

Ten

SUN SALUTATIONS—SURYA NAMASKAR
(SIR-yah nah-mah-SCAR)

Turn your face to the sun and the shadows fall behind you.
—Maori proverb

For many ages in India this series of flowing Yoga poses has been performed in the early morning, facing the rising sun, as a moving prayer and a way to greet the day. The series came to be known as the Sun Salutation. *Surya* means "sun" and *namaskar* means "greeting" or "salutation."

The Sun Salutation is the best-known series of movements in yoga. I learned them in my very first yoga class back in 1971, and I have taught them as part of every class I have given. I love them and do them nearly every day. I start my morning practice with at least a dozen repetitions of the Sun Salutation. During the first few repetitions I feel stiff, but after doing several Sun Salutations, flexibility returns; it feels so good to stretch. I often perform Sun Salutations quickly, which generates heat and creates a cardiovascular workout. It is also wonderful to do them slowly as a deliberate way to release tightness and muscular tension.

Sun Salutations are a great way to stretch every part of the body. They tone the abdominal organs and reduce abdominal fat, improve spinal flexibility, aid good posture, and increase circulation. They have a positive effect on the cardiovascular and cardiopulmonary systems. Sun

Salutations are also an excellent way to relieve tension and promote relaxation.

CAUTION: Do not do the Sun Salutations if you have unmanaged high blood pressure, a herniated disk, or are suffering from acute sciatica.

Sun Salutations can be used at any time in a yoga class. In the Gentle Stretch Yoga, we do them toward the end of the class after practicing the other yoga poses and just before doing deep relaxation. Because they demand effort and stamina, Sun Salutations make lying down in the Relaxation Pose all the more welcome.

There are many variations of Sun Salutations but all consist of a series of poses, usually twelve, that flow together in a sequential order. The movements alternate from a forward-bending to a backward-bending movement of the spine. The first five poses are the same as the last five in opposite order, with poses six and seven varying in the degree of difficulty and intensity.

If you are learning the Sun Salutations, it will be helpful to break down the series into the individual poses. Familiarize yourself with each pose and then move through them as part of a sequence.

Once you know the sequence of poses, add the breathing instructions. Inhale in each movement where you stretch up or expand your chest and exhale as you bend forward. Your coordination of your breath with each movement ensures regular breathing, provides a steady and pleasant rhythm to the Sun Salutations, and is beneficial in increasing lung capacity. If using one breath per movement causes you to move more quickly than feels comfortable, take the breaths you need in each of the positions.

How to Use a Chair in the Sun Salutations

Using a chair to perform the Sun Salutations provides an advantage for a body that is stiff or tight. This adaptation helps my oldest students make it through many cycles of the series with relative ease. By adding a chair to the Sun Salutations, you raise the floor up eighteen inches higher, and that makes each forward and backward bend easier to perform and less intense. The chair may be the means for you to change this series of poses from impossible to manageable or easy. That is the case for Ted, a gentleman in his seventies, who demonstrates the Sun Salutations with a chair in the following instructions.

SUN SALUTATION WITH A CHAIR

If you have a yoga mat, put your mat on the floor, and place your chair at one end of the mat with the seat of the chair facing into the mat. Make sure that all four legs of the chair are on the mat to prevent the chair from slipping.

If you do not have a yoga mat, place the back of your chair against a wall or a heavy piece of furniture so that your chair won't move. This is imperative for your safety. Without a nonslip mat beneath your chair, and nothing to brace the chair against, your chair could slip as you lean into it, and so could you.

Stand facing the seat of the chair, with your feet slightly apart. Line up the tops of your toes even with the front legs of the chair.

Begin in Mountain Pose. Be still and quiet. Observe yourself while you take a couple of deep breaths in and out. You are ready to begin.

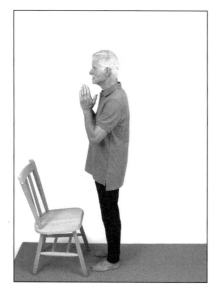

Sun Salutation with a Chair, Position 1

Position 1

Sun Salutation with a Chair, Position 1

Place the palms and fingers of your hands together in a prayer position in front of your chest with your thumbs resting lightly on your breastbone.

Exhale slowly.

Position 2

Sun Salutation with a Chair, Position 2

Raise your arms overhead as you breathe in.

Allow your palms to separate. Keep your arms strong, straight, and parallel.

Stretch and look up. (For those with a weak lower back, bend your knees slightly to take pressure off your lower back and then stretch up.)

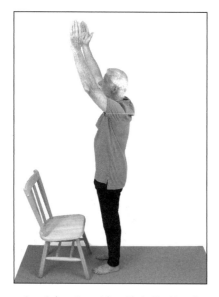

Sun Salutation with a Chair, Position 2

Position 3

Sun Salutation with a Chair, Position 3

Breathe out as you fold forward from the hips.

Bring your hands to either side of the chair seat or, alternatively, onto the front edge of the chair. Try both variations of hand placement on the chair to see which is most comfortable for your wrists in this position and for all the others.

Touch your head to the seat of the chair if you can. If you have to bend your knees and round your back to do this, that's fine.

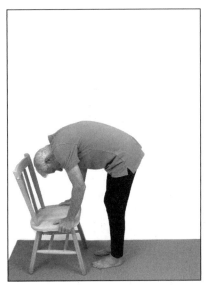

Sun Salutation with a Chair, Position 3

Position 4

Sun Salutation with a Chair, Position 4

Lift your head as you inhale and step your right foot back as far as you can.

Bend your left knee until it touches the chair.

Lower your hips toward the chair.

Press your hands against the chair, lift your chest, stretch, and look up.

Move your shoulders down and away from your ears.

Press your back heel down toward the ground to get a good stretch in the back of your lower leg. Your back heel will not be able to reach the floor, so don't try to force it.

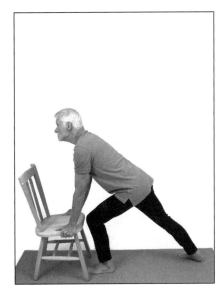

Sun Salutation with a Chair, Position 4

SUN SALUTATIONS

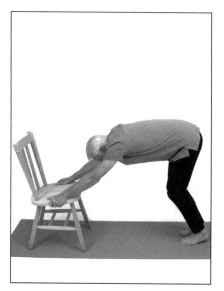

Sun Salutation with a Chair, Position 5

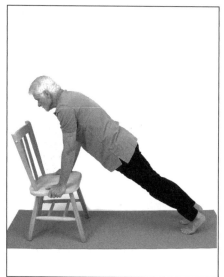

Sun Salutation with a Chair, Position 6

Position 5

Sun Salutation with a Chair, Position 5

This is the chair version of Downward-Facing Dog Pose.

Move your left foot back in line with your right foot as you exhale, with your feet about 6 to 8 inches apart.

Push back from your hands on the chair. Move your buttocks back as far from the chair as you can, stretching the extension of your spine. Bend your knees if the backs of your legs are tight to get the maximum length and extension of your spine.

Keep your arms straight and lower your head between your arms.

Look down at the floor.

Position 6

Sun Salutation with a Chair, Position 6

This pose is a weight-bearing position for your arms and one that helps to strengthen your arms and wrists.

Come up onto the balls of your feet as you move your body weight forward onto your arms.

Drop your hips down to make your body completely straight.

Lift your torso up from your arms, rather than collapsing down and allowing your shoulders to move up toward your ears.

Breathe in and stay in this position through position 7 if you have a lower-back weakness or injury.

●

Position 7

CAUTION: Do not do this movement if you have lower-back weakness or injury. Instead, skip this movement and go on to position 8.

Sun Salutation with a Chair, Position 7

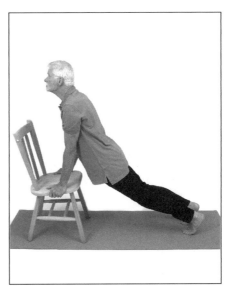

Sun Salutation with a Chair, Position 7

Through the inhalation in the previous position, continue to move your hips closer toward the chair, as you push up and away from your hands. Arch your back and stretch as you look up.

●

Position 8

Sun Salutation with a Chair, Position 8

Repeat position 5

As you exhale, push your hips back away from the chair. Push back from your hands and extend your spine as much as you can.

Move your buttocks as far away from the chair as possible.

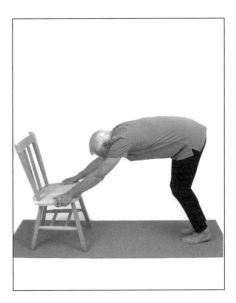

Sun Salutation with a Chair, Position 8

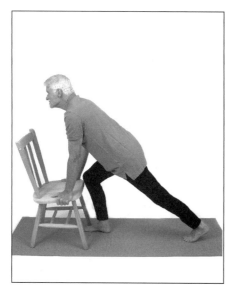

Sun Salutation with a Chair, Position 9

Position 9

Sun Salutation with a Chair, Position 9

Repeat position 4 with the opposite leg forward
    As you breathe in, bring your right foot forward
to the chair.
    Bend your knee to touch the seat of the chair.
Don't forget to lower your hips down as you lift
your chest and look up.

Position 10

Sun Salutation with a Chair, Position 10

Step forward to the chair with your left leg.
    Bend forward and lower your head to the seat of
the chair (if you can) as you exhale all your breath.

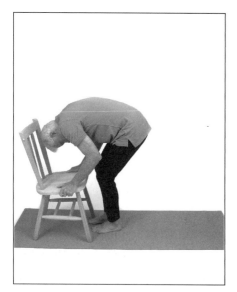

Sun Salutation with a Chair, Position 10

YOGA FOR ALL OF US

Position 11

Sun Salutation with a Chair, Position 11

Raise your head, your upper body, and lift your arms overhead as you breathe in.

Stretch up, bring your palms together, and look up.

Position 12

Sun Salutation with a Chair, Position 12

Keep your palms together, exhale slowly, and lower your arms.

Bring your palms to the front of your chest.

This completes the sequence.

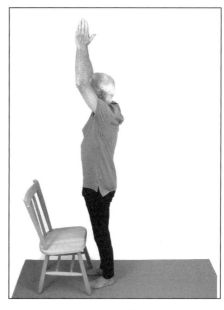

Sun Salutation with a Chair, Position 11

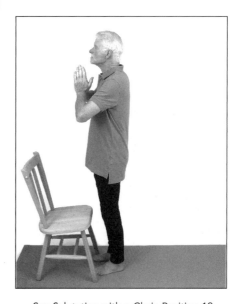

Sun Salutation with a Chair, Position 12

Do the Sun Salutations that follow without the chair if your hips are flexible and your body moves with ease. If you try this and find it too strenuous or difficult, then learn the chair variation. You benefit most by selecting whichever form works best for your body at this time. But if you already know the Sun Salutations, I encourage you to try the chair version also. Some of the positions from the chair stretch the body differently than those on the floor. I often start my morning yoga practice using the chair for the first few repetitions of Sun Salutations. When I have loosened up and am more flexible, I continue the Sun Salutations using the traditional method. This approach eases me into a comfortable and enjoyable experience.

●

Position 1

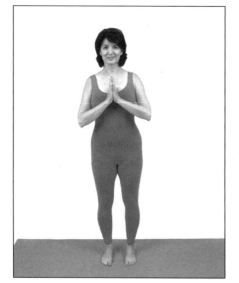

Stand in Mountain Pose at the top of your mat (if you are using a mat).

Sun Salutation Position 1, Front View

Place the palms and fingers of your hands together in a prayer position in front of your chest with your thumbs resting lightly on your breastbone.
   Exhale slowly.

Sun Salutation Position 1, Front View

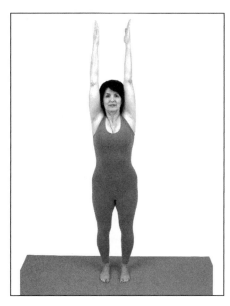

Sun Salutation Position 2, Front View

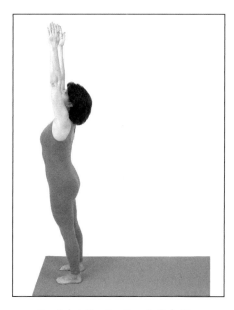

Sun Salutation Position 2, Side View

Position 2

Sun Salutation Position 2, Front View and Side View

Raise your arms overhead as you breathe in.

Stretch and look up. (For those with a weak lower back, bend your knees slightly to take pressure off your lower back and then stretch up.)

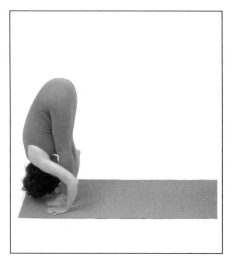

Sun Salutation Position 3

Position 3

Sun Salutation, Position 3

Breathe out slowly as you lower your arms, and bend your torso forward from the hips.

Keep your spine straight and extended as you bend forward.

Bring your hands to either side of your feet, aligning your fingertips with your toes. (You may have to bend your knees to do this.)

Position 4

Sun Salutation, Position 4

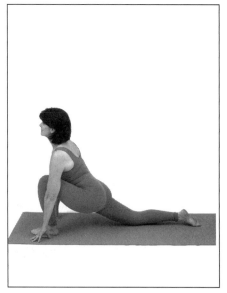

Sun Salutation, Position 4

As you inhale, step your right foot back as far as you can.

Lower your hips toward the floor as you bend your left knee into a lunge position.

Drop your back knee to the floor, or leave your back leg straight with your knee lifted off the floor.

Lift your chest and head up. Come up onto your fingertips if this gives you a better stretch and enables you to lift out of your shoulders.

YOGA FOR ALL OF US

Position 5

Sun Salutation, Position 5

As you exhale, bring your left foot back to the right foot, placing it so that your feet are 6 to 8 inches apart. This is Downward-Facing Dog position.

Spread your fingers wide apart. Place your hands so that your middle fingers point directly forward.

Press your hands into the floor and push back firmly from your hands and arms. Keep your arms straight and strong.

Move your head between your arms, aligning your neck with your spine.

If the backs of your legs are tight, bend your knees. Keep your knees bent and lift your buttocks up toward the ceiling to create a long extension in your spine.

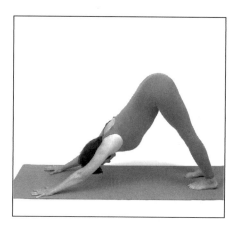

Sun Salutation, Position 5

Position 6

Sun Salutation, Position 6

Move your body weight forward, shifting your weight to your arms.

Lower your hips until your entire body is as straight as a plank, known as the Plank Pose.

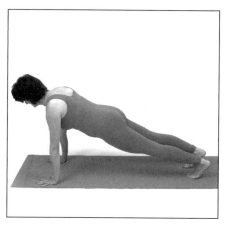

Sun Salutation, Position 6

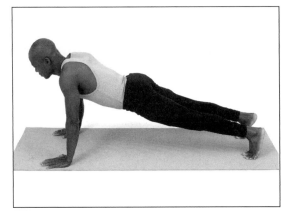

Sun Salutation Position 6, Kwame in Plank Pose

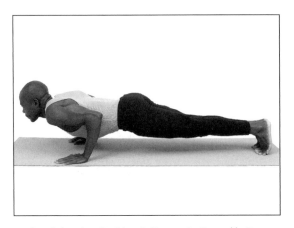

Sun Salutation Position 6, Kwame in Crocodile Pose

SUN SALUTATION ADVANCED VARIATION (OPTIONAL)

Sun Salutation Position 6, Kwame in Plank Pose

Move to plank pose.

Sun Salutation Position 6, Kwame in Crocodile Pose

Lower yourself to a push-up position, known as Crocodile Pose.

Position 7

CAUTION: Do not do this position if you have concerns about the strength of your back. Instead, skip this position and go to position 8.

Sun Salutation Position 7, Kwame on the Tops of the Feet

Move your hips forward and down toward the floor as you push up and away from your hands.

Lift your chest, stretch upward, and look up as you breathe in.

You can have your feet in two positions on the tops of the feet or . . .

Sun Salutation, Position 7, on Toes

You can remain on your toes.

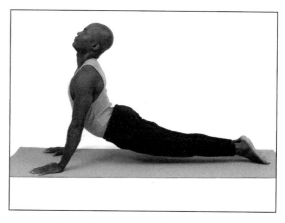

Sun Salutation Position 7, Kwame on the Tops of the Feet

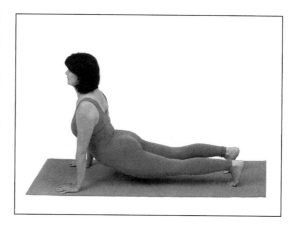

Sun Salutation, Position 7

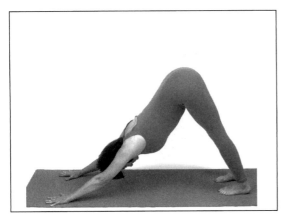

Sun Salutation, Position 8

Position 8

Move your hips back and up as you exhale and return to position 5, Downward-Facing Dog Pose.

Sun Salutation, Position 8

Push away from your hands, keeping your arms firm.

Extend your spine as much as you can, lifting your buttocks up to the ceiling.

Position 9

Progression from position 8 to 9 is the most difficult movement of any in the Sun Salutation. If your right foot does not easily move up all the way between your hands, take hold of your right ankle and physically move that foot into position either with one big step or in a series of smaller steps.

Sun Salutation, Position 9

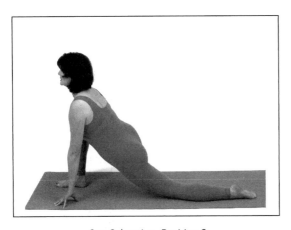

Sun Salutation, Position 9

As you breathe in, bring your right foot forward into a lunge, which is position 4, with the opposite leg forward.

Open your chest and pull your shoulders back as you look up and extend your spine.

YOGA FOR ALL OF US

Position 10

Sun Salutation, Position 10

Repeat position 3. Step forward with your left leg, bringing your left foot in line with your right. Keep 6 to 8 inches of space between your feet.

Bring your head as close to your lower legs as you can. (You can bend your knees and round your back.)

Exhale completely.

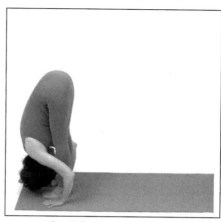

Sun Salutation, Position 10

Position 11

Sun Salutation Position 11, Side View and Front View

Repeat position 2, bringing your palms together overhead.

As you inhale, raise your head, upper body, and arms.

Return to an upright position.

Stretch up as you look up.

Bring your palms together overhead.

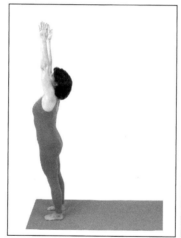

Sun Salutation Position 11, Front View

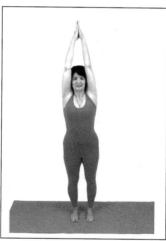

Sun Salutation Position 11, Side View

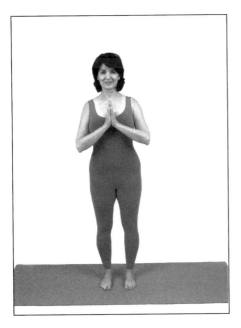

Sun Salutation Position 12, Front View

Position 12

Sun Salutation Position 12, Front View

Exhale and lower your palms down to the middle of your chest. You are back where you started the sequence, in position 1.

The flow of these twelve poses makes up one Sun Salutation. That is one-half of a full round of Sun Salutations.

In the second half of the round, alternate the movement of your legs, stepping back with the left leg in position 4 rather than the right one. In position 9, your left leg moves forward instead of your right. Two Sun Salutation (the first one moving your right leg, and the second moving your left leg) makes one round. Practicing the Sun Salutation as a round provides a balanced and even stretch for each leg.

Start with three rounds. I call that the DMR—the Daily Minimum Requirement for Sun Salutations. Once you are doing these three comfortably, you may want to add more rounds to your practice.

You may want to keep track of the number of rounds that you are doing (although this is not necessary to your practice). Here is one way to remember how many you have done.

Each time you begin a new round, say out loud the number of the round you are on. If you hear yourself say the number out loud, you reinforce your memory of that number better than by just keeping track of the number silently.

I have also devised a counting system that is a more active and visual

YOGA FOR ALL OF US

method. Take ten coins and place them to the back left corner on the seat of your chair, if you are using a chair for your Sun Salutations. If not, place the coins on the floor near the upper left corner of your mat.

After completing each round, move a coin from the left corner to the right one. When all ten coins have been moved, you have completed ten rounds or twenty Sun Salutations.

One other method of doing a similar number of rounds consistently over time: find a piece of music you enjoy, one with a steady and even beat, like Pachelbel's *Canon in D* that I use in class. Build up the number of Sun Salutations until you are doing them through the whole piece of music. Then each time you play that music while doing your Sun Salutations, you have a set and consistent length of time to perform them.

My teacher, Swami Muktananda, used to say that, with time, everyone could work up to doing one hundred Sun Salutations a day. If you move quickly enough, you can do one hundred repetitions in a little over twenty minutes. That's five a minute or one (consisting of the twelve poses) in twelve seconds. That is literally one pose per second. At that pace the Sun Salutations are definitely a cardiovascular workout.

Long ago there was a king in the Maharashtra state in India who popularized the practice of Sun Salutations by performing one thousand a day! It takes about three hours to do that many repetitions, but if you do that many, it's fair to say you don't need to do any other yoga to maintain health.

No matter how many Sun Salutations you do, they provide more benefit than running or jogging for the same amount of time. This is great news for runners who have injured their knees or feet and can no longer run.

There are few people who desire ever attempting doing one hundred Sun Salutations in one session (fifty rounds). But if you would like to challenge yourself and build up to that number, do it the gentle way. Start with three or five rounds and add an additional round every day. At that pace you will reach the goal of one hundred repetitions before two months pass.

Eleven

RELAXATION

The time to relax is when you don't have time for it.
—Sidney J. Harris, newspaper columnist

At the end of a yoga practice, no matter how long or short, make Relaxation Pose your final pose. If you only have time to do a few yoga poses each day, include Relaxation Pose. If time is short, people often think they can skip this pose at the end of their practice because it seems as if nothing is happening in this pose. But "nothing" is just what makes this pose so valuable. As you lie in the relaxation pose, the body destresses—breathing slows and becomes even and steady, blood pressure lowers, and brain waves change rhythm. That is why after the end of practice, words like calm, peaceful, quiet, centered, even blissful may best describe your state of being.

When you take the time to do the relaxation pose at the end of your practice, you take full advantage of the effects of all the preceding yoga poses. As you lie down in a way that is stretched out and open, your circulation, both that of your blood and your subtle energy currents, flows unrestricted to all parts of your body. A fresh supply of oxygen and nutrients flows into each cell and accumulated toxins and impurities are released to be eliminated from the body. The subtle current of your *prana* (life force) is distributed to your organs, glands, tissues, nerves, and cells; and because of this, the systems of the body are invigorated and balanced.

I guarantee that at the end of practicing yoga poses, including the Relaxation Pose, you will feel better than when you started. If you do nothing else, Relaxation Pose is valuable on its own.

I refer to this pose as the Relaxation Pose, but its name in Sanskrit means "corpse" and is often called Corpse Pose. The instructions in a seventeenth-century manual on yoga, the *Gheranda-Samhita*, describe the pose as "lying flat on the ground like a corpse" (see Georg Feuerstein, *The Shambhala Encyclopedia of Yoga,* Shambhala Publications, 1997, pp. 105, 188, 276). The challenge of this pose is simply to lie down as if you were dead. It means getting your body completely still, free from muscular tension, and totally relaxed. The challenge doesn't end there because usually, when we lie down and are quiet and still, we go to sleep.

In Relaxation Pose you are not looking for sleep. The goal in the Relaxation Pose is to keep your mind awake and focused, while you relax your body even more completely than when you are sound asleep. In the beginning it may be difficult to stay awake when you are so deeply relaxed, especially if you are tired or sleep deprived. Don't worry if you do drift off. If you do, know that you probably needed the extra sleep. In time you will develop an ability to remain conscious while you relax deeply. It takes practice, but the rewards are extraordinary.

●

RELAXATION POSE—SAVASANA (SHAH-VAHS-ANNA)

To ensure success when you perform Relaxation Pose:

Choose a quiet place where you will be undisturbed for at least 5 to 10 minutes. If you have the time, I recommend setting aside 10 minutes so you won't have to "hurry" to relax.

Relaxation Pose, Head and Knee Support

Set a timer so that you don't have to open your eyes to check your watch or worry about the time if you think that you may drift off to sleep.

Use pillows underneath your head and knees if that makes you more comfortable.

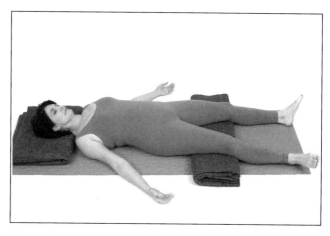

Relaxation Pose, Head and Knee Support

Relaxation Pose, Lower Legs on Chair, Yoga Student Ted

If you have lower back discomfort, you may benefit by modifying the Relaxation Pose. Place your lower legs on the seat of a chair; this bent-knee position further supports and relaxes your back muscles.

Cover yourself with a blanket if you get chilled easily. The body

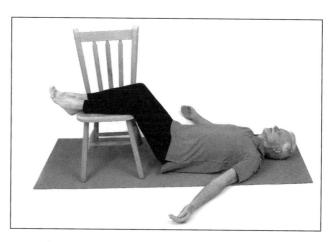

Relaxation Pose, Lower Legs on Chair, Yoga Student Ted

cools down rapidly as you relax, which is why we use blankets at night when we sleep.

Set an intention of total relaxation by thinking, "Now I am going to relax." An intention helps focus your mind and clearly states what you want.

RELAXATION

The relaxation begins with suggestions for your overall relaxation and is followed by detailed and specific instructions in three steps:

Step 1. Focuses on relaxation of your facial muscles: eyes, forehead, cheeks, jaw, and lips.

Step 2. Includes the rest of your head and your neck, shoulders, arms, and hands.

Step 3. Moves the relaxation through your torso, hips, legs, and feet. Finally, you expand your awareness to include your entire body.

Relaxation Pose

Lie down on your back with your legs a little apart and your arms a little away from your sides with your palms facing up.

Lift your head to check your body's alignment. Make sure that your feet are evenly spaced apart and your arms are angled away from your torso an equal distance. Lower your head and close your eyes.

Bring your attention to your breathing. Practice the belly breathing and make your breaths slow, deep, and even.

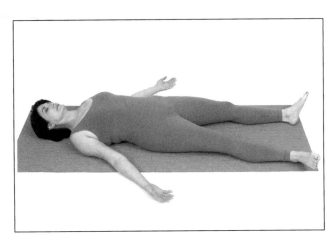

Relaxation Pose

Step 1. Relax the muscles of your face.

Become aware of the muscles of your face and relax them.

Close your eyes and focus your attention on your eye muscles.

Soften the area around your eyes. Relax your eye muscles until they feel so comfortable that all tension and tightness around your eyes seems to melt away.

YOGA FOR ALL OF US

Imagine that your eyelids are very heavy and totally relaxed, so relaxed that it would be difficult to open them.

Imagine the relaxation that you have created in your eye muscles spreading up to your forehead and down to your cheeks . . . and into your jaw . . . and to your lips.

As your lips and jaw relax, your lips will gently separate, and you can use this as a sign that you are bringing about deep relaxation in your facial muscles.

Imagine all the muscles of your face as very soft and smooth.

Step 2. Relax the muscles of your head, neck, shoulders, arms, and hands.

From the top of your head, imagine that you send a wave of relaxation down the back of your head, which causes the tiny scalp muscles to relax.

Send this wave of relaxation into your neck, softening those muscles . . . and then down into your shoulders.

Spend a few moments aware of the muscles of the neck and shoulders and releasing any tightness.

Spread the relaxation out through your shoulders and down into your arms.

Let your arms become completely limp and loose. Take your time.

Continue the flow of relaxation through your wrists and into your hands and fingers.

Step 3. Relax the muscles of your torso, legs, and feet.

From your shoulders, send the relaxation into your chest . . . stomach area . . . and down to your hips.

Also from your shoulders, send the relaxation into your back muscles, the muscles along your spine, and your lower back and buttocks.

From your hips, send the relaxation out into your legs . . . through your ankles to your feet and toes.

Return your awareness to your entire body.

Imagine letting go even more, and double the level of your relaxation.

Keep your awareness on your body as a whole as you experience "yogic sleep." You will be awake, aware, very comfortable, and relaxed.

When you hear your alarm, or are ready to return to your regular activities, do not leap from the floor back into activity. Be gentle with yourself as you bring yourself to your waking consciousness.

Gently move your fingers and toes.

Stretch your limbs.

Pull your knees into your chest.

Roll over to your right side.

Push yourself with your hands up to an upright position.

Spend a few moments reorienting yourself in an upright position as you take stock of how you feel.

Twelve

MEDITATION, EXERCISES FOR YOUR MIND

If we have not quiet in our minds, outward comfort will do no
more for us than a golden slipper on a gouty foot.
—John Bunyan (1628–88) English preacher and writer

Meditation has incredible physical, mental, and spiritual benefits for
both the short and long term. Meditation is not an end in itself; it
is a journey and a process. No one sits down and does it right the first
time or the hundredth time because there actually is no right way to do
it.

Meditation is an important part of each Gentle Stretch Yoga Class I
teach, and it is the first thing we do. It is part of my day, every day, and
has been for thirty-five years. I know that there are many misconcep-
tions about meditation, just as there are about yoga. Just as you don't
have to contort yourself to do yoga poses, you don't have to be a monk
to meditate. There are some easy and helpful steps to help you learn to
meditate. After the Meditation Exercises, I will give you additional information and hints to help you continue your meditation practice.

Although there is no right method of meditation, there are some specific and helpful ways to meditate based on hundreds of years of practice. Read these instructions to make your first experience easier.

WHY MEDITATE?

The rewards of meditation are tremendous. Meditation produces measurable results in addition to subjective effects. International research on meditation documents the positive physiological effect of meditation—blood pressure is lowered naturally, respiration slows, breathing deepens, stress hormones decrease, muscular tension eases, and brain activity slows down. In addition to recognized physical changes, meditation yields personal benefits. It lightens your spirit, calms your mind, and reduces emotional turmoil. All these effects contribute to the enhanced immune system functioning that is essential for healing or preventing disease.

WHAT IS MEDITATION?

Meditation is a method of bringing your attention to the present moment rather than thinking about the past or future. Meditation evidences a willingness to look at and be with "what is," and provides an opportunity to detach yourself from your customary reactions and judgments. Meditation is a process of redirecting your thinking to subdue your mental chatter so you can experience an inner source of knowing and a place of profound peace and clarity. Through regular meditation you gain a different perspective on who you are.

Meditation is a way of quieting the body and mind so that your mind has an opportunity to slow down and take a break. Short-term results are that you simply sit still for a few minutes in your busy day. The long-term outcome and benefits you experience will change and multiply toward an expanded consciousness.

HOW TO MEDITATE

There are many forms of meditation from all over the world. Most approaches use a focus for your awareness: On the breath, a special word or a mantra (a sacred word or phrase, you have probably heard the word "om" used), a sound or a visual object. Another form of meditation is mindfulness of thinking, the development of awareness of what the mind is thinking without getting involved in the content of the thought. I will give you six specific meditation exercises to try.

Because meditation is training for your mind, it is important to keep the structure of it uniform and consistent. Set aside a time for meditation, ideally the same time every day. Take time immediately after waking, before the hectic daily schedule begins, or make time at a natural break in your day—after coming home from work, at lunchtime, or anytime that has a natural pace change.

Once you have chosen your time, make it a regular part of each day. Make an appointment with yourself for meditation. By doing this you give meditation a special place in your day and in your life and are less likely to skip meditation on any day.

If the idea of sitting in one place for long seems difficult, start by sitting to meditate for as little as ten minutes of quiet for the first couple of weeks. As that time period becomes comfortable, increase your meditation time to twenty minutes at a stretch. When you choose a specific amount of time to meditate, like a twenty minute period, commit to that designated amount of time rather than taking twenty minutes one day, fifteen the next, and twenty-five the day after that. Be intentional and consistent about the amount of time you practice each session. Your body and your mind will come to accept your chosen time period and settle in more readily. You can set a timer to sound at the end of the time period so that you free yourself from having to check your watch or guessing how long you have been meditating.

Choose a regular place to practice, preferably one free from distractions and disturbance. If you have the space, make it a special place of its own. When you come to sit there, your body and mind will know "this is the time and place for meditation."

As you start to practice and experiment with the exercises in meditation,

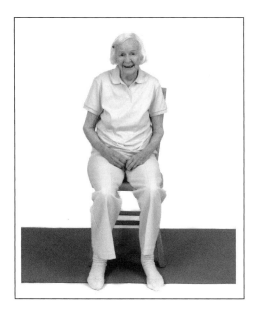

Chair Position for Meditation, Yoga Student Jo

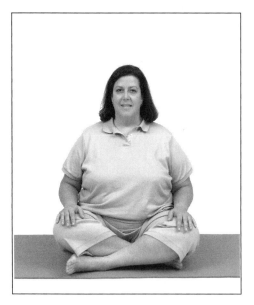

Cross-legged Pose for Meditation, Yoga Student Cathie

you may feel restless or bored. Don't give up and get up. Don't think *Nothing is happening.* Watch your reactions with curiosity and interest. Make your success in meditation not about how long you remain focused or thought free, or what you "see" or don't see. Make your success a willingness to persevere and sit for your intended time; and whenever your mind wanders, bring it back to your object of focus.

Choose your position for meditation; either sit in a chair or take a traditional seated position on the floor. If you want to sit in a chair, choose a firm one, a chair that does not offer the opportunity to slump so you can keep your spine straight and tall. It is easier to meditate when you are balanced, comfortable, and relaxed. In the Gentle Stretch Yoga Class, we meditate while seated in a chair, and this is what I recommend if you are not used to or comfortable sitting on the floor.

If you sit on the floor, use the Cross-legged Pose (see page 146) if you are not familiar with another seated position for meditation. Remember, it is helpful to sit on a firm pillow or folded blanket so that your hips are raised higher than your knees to help you keep your spine straight. Place your cushion on a soft surface like a carpet, pad, or blanket to reduce the pressure of the floor against your feet. If it is difficult to keep your back upright and relaxed in this position, sit with your back against a wall or piece of immovable furniture. If you have

YOGA FOR ALL OF US

knee problems, you can extend one or both legs out in front of you.

If you have a physical limitation that prevents you from sitting up-right, you can practice meditation from a reclining position. Use Savasana, the Relaxation Pose (see page 173). The major disadvantage of lying down for meditation is that you may be too comfortable and fall asleep. With practice, however, you will become better at staying present and aware while in the Relaxation Pose.

To Begin Your Meditation

The first two exercises will help to focus you and heighten your aware-ness of yourself and your breathing. Start with either of these two or both. Then add whichever of the other exercises that is most appealing for the remainder of the time.

When you meditate, close your eyes and relax the muscles around your eyes. If you want to keep your eyes open, rest them in a relaxed way on one spot to decrease surrounding visual stimuli. It is the nature of your senses to perceive external stimulation, and since meditation is an "interiorization," a process of turning inward, it is helpful to limit visual input.

●

Meditation 1: Focus on Your Body

Choose your seated position, either in a chair or on the floor. Rest your hands in your lap or on your thighs. Close your eyes. Start this way for this and all of the meditations to follow.

Become aware of the places that your body makes contact with the floor and/or the support of the chair.

In the Cross-legged Pose, feel the floor (or pillow or blanket) against your buttocks, thighs, and feet.

In a chair with your feet on the floor, feel the pressure of the floor against the bottoms of your feet. Feel the chair against your buttocks, thighs, and back.

Stay still and aware for a few breaths.

Feel the pressure of your hands where they rest on your thighs.

Become aware of the sensation of your clothing against your skin, as well as eyeglasses, a watch, or any jewelry you may be wearing. Many people choose to remove their eyeglasses for meditation. Chances are it will be difficult to detect your watch or jewelry if you are accustomed to wearing it.

Expand your awareness to be conscious of all of the above at the same time.

Return your awareness to these sensations whenever you catch your mind wandering to another topic. By focusing on these sensations, you bring your mind out of the everyday concerns and into a less hurried state.

●

Meditation 2: Focus on Your Breath

Become aware of your breathing and follow your inhalations and exhalations. Breath through your nose if possible.

Examine the quality of your breathing:

Are your inhalations and exhalations equal in length?

Is your breathing smooth or does it catch, is it even or rough and uneven?

Is your breathing fast or slow, shallow or deep?

Notice the point of entry and exit of your breath at your nostrils.

Is there a temperature difference between the inhalation and the exhalation?

Notice the space or pause between each breath as it turns inward or outward.

Be aware of the movement in your chest and/or belly as you breathe in and out.

By adding this focus on your breathing, your mind has another level of sensation to focus on that will bring it out of thinking of the past or the future and into the present "now." These two preceding exercises are a good way to start a meditation session. Add one of the following meditations to complete the amount of time you have promised yourself.

●

Meditation 3: Counting Your Breaths

Make your breathing slower and deeper.

Count each breath, inhalation and exhalation, together as one count.

Count from 1 to 10. If you lose track of the number you are on, either start again at 1 or pick up counting from the last number you remember.

Once you reach 10, begin again from 1 and count to 10 again. Or count backward from 10 to 1.

●

Meditation 4: Recite a Short Verse with Your Breath

The Vietnamese monk, Thich Nhat Hanh, is a respected and honored teacher who has written many books on meditation and "mindfulness," the process of being aware of what you are experiencing while aware of yourself as the experiencer. He says it is helpful to recite a short verse, like the ones below, to remind yourself of what is going on.

Say to yourself as you breathe in, "I know I am breathing in," or simply "In."

Say to yourself as you breathe out, "I know I am breathing out," or simply "Out."

You can add other phrases like:

"As I breathe in, I calm myself," or "Calm."
"As I breathe out, I release tension," or "Releasing tension."

After a couple of minutes linking your breath and a phrase, finish with:

"I am aware of the present moment," or "Present moment," as you breathe in.
"I am aware that it is a wonderful moment," or "Wonderful moment," as you breath out.

Meditation 5: Use a Mantra or Special Word

A mantra is a sacred word, spiritual phrase, or name of God. "Man" means "to think" and "tra" means "instrumental"; "mantra" literally means "instrument of thought." The repeated use of a mantra is designed to connect you with higher consciousness.

The best known Sanskrit mantra is "Om," which is considered to be the primordial vibration of creation or the "sound of all sounds." Om is often chanted at the beginning and end of a yoga practice to evoke the Divine or one's higher power.

For this exercise, use "Hamsa" (hum sah), a mantra that was given to me by my meditation teacher, Swami Muktananda. "Hamsa" is considered to be the sound of the natural rhythm of the breath. When you breathe deeply and are aware of and "present" with your breath, you can hear "hamsa" deep within. It is called the mantra of the "Self" and can be easily repeated by people of any faith or religion.

Say to yourself "Ham (hum)" as you breathe in.
Say to yourself "sa (sah)" as you breathe out.

If you prefer, you can choose any sacred word to use in this exercise, for example, "Amen," or, use a simple, uplifting word like "Love." If you use a special word instead of "Hamsa," say it to yourself during each breath in and each breath out.

Follow your breath with the mantra or your chosen word. Whenever you find yourself thinking other thoughts, lead your mind back to the repetition of the mantra.

●

Meditation 6: Focus on a Visual Object

Choose an object such as a flower, a piece of fruit, a candle, or a stone.

Keep your eyes open and softly focused on your object. When you realize that you are thinking of other things, return your mind to your object of meditation.

Option: Close your eyes and make a mental picture of your object. Reopen them to include more details, then close your eyes again and stay focused on your mental image.

●

To End Your Meditation

When your timer rings or your set time for meditation has ended, do not immediately get up.

Bring your awareness to yourself breathing.

Open your eyes.

Notice your surroundings.

Take a moment to experience your mental and emotional state.

Mentally acknowledge yourself for taking the time you did and set the intention for meditation again tomorrow.

Then stretch your limbs, massage your legs and ankles if you have been sitting on the floor, and return to your normal activity.

Now that you have practiced a meditation you may be wondering how you did. If you sat for your intended amount of time and you tried to focus on the breathing and the sensations, then you did just fine. It is unfortunate that in the United States there is such an intense emphasis on doing things right. Just as there is no right or wrong way to meditate—what is important is that you simply observe your inner and outer reality without judging them—there is also no best kind of experience to have while meditating. Sometimes your mind will race with thoughts; at other times you'll remember things you have forgotten. You may feel very calm and quiet, drowsy or sleepy, or so energized you want to leap up and do something. You might see images with your eyes closed, hear inner sounds, or perceive unfamiliar bodily sensations like falling or floating. None of these experiences is to be sought, and each experience of meditation will be different.

The aim of meditation is to quiet your thoughts or heighten your awareness of yourself in the present moment. Don't assume that when your mind does become quiet that you will have no more thoughts the next time you meditate. It is the nature of the mind to think. The meditation exercises help train your mind how to deal with ever-present and run-away thoughts. With practice, you may notice an increased ability to quiet your mind through meditation and an experience of peace. In the meantime, when you find your mind going off to your grocery list or an upcoming appointment, don't get upset; gently bring your focus back to the object of meditation you have chosen.

There is a spiritual component to meditation because meditation connects you to your own deeper being and moves you into a state of greater awareness. It can serve as a connection with the divine. However, there is nothing specifically religious about meditation, and people of all faiths and denominations practice it in harmony with their own religious practices. While meditation is a way to calm and quiet the mind, as well as rest the body, it is above all a way to experience yourself in a greater and more profound way and through that to more fully un-

YOGA FOR ALL OF US

derstand what life is all about.

The benefits of meditation that have been documented by both the medical and spiritual communities result from a peaceful body and a quiet mind. Even if you don't think that you are getting a quiet mind or any connection you can identify between your mind and body, I encourage you to keep trying and don't give up. If you try meditation for at least a month, just like doing the yoga poses regularly, you will see a difference in yourself. Your experience of meditation will grow and expand. All the great meditation teachers have left us with this encouragement: Go within and discover your invisible higher self.

> Let us then labor for an inward stillness,—
> An inward stillness and an inward healing,
> That perfect silence when the lips and heart
> Are still,
> and we no longer entertain
> Our own imperfect thoughts. . . .
> —Henry Wadsworth Longfellow (1807–82)
> American poet and educator

NAMASTE

I honor that Greatness that dwells within you as you.
—Peggy Cappy

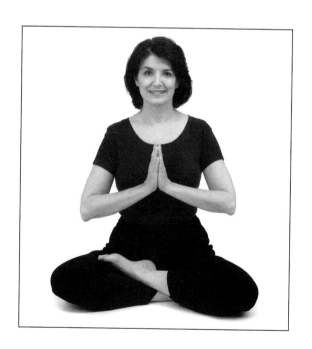

INDEX

INDEX

INDEX